D0195068

NOURISH
&
GLOW

ALSO BY JULES ARON

Zen and Tonic: Savory and Fresh Cocktails for the Enlightened Drinker

Vegan Cheese: Simple, Delicious, Plant-Based Recipes

Fresh & Pure: Organically Crafted Beauty Balms & Cleansers

NOURISH
&
GLOW

Naturally Beautifying
Foods & Elixirs

Jules Aron

THE COUNTRYMAN PRESS
A division of W. W. Norton & Company
Independent Publishers Since 1923

33614080554016

To my loving parents,
who instilled in me, in equal doses,
a great love and appreciation for good food
and the importance of taking responsibility
for your own health.

And to all of you passionate foodies,
here's to living each day with the freedom
to choose what's right for you
and to supporting each other
in the global shift to a healthier,
more beautiful world.

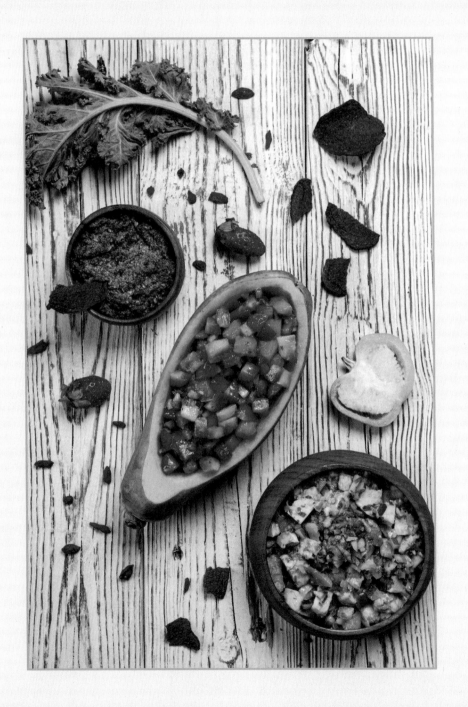

CONTENTS

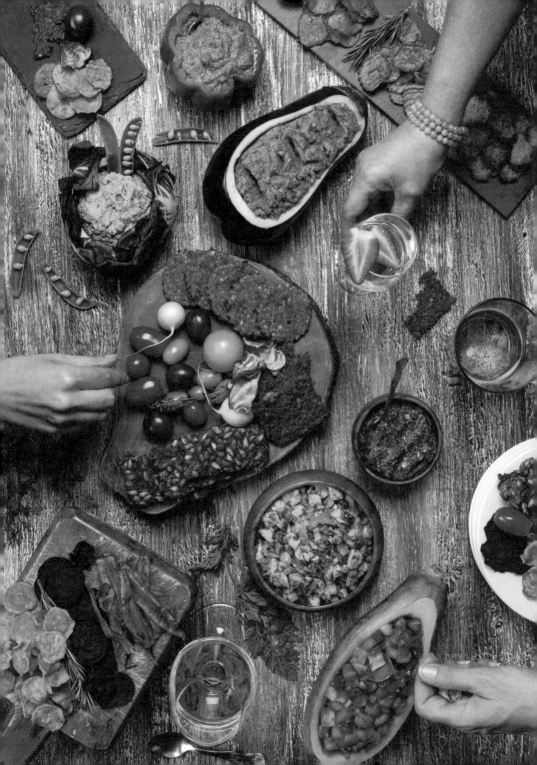

INTRODUCTION

*A life of beauty begins one nourishing
meal at a time.*

I grew up around the kitchen table. For my family, food was everything. My father owned and managed several restaurants, while my mom worked as a chef in some of the most prestigious international hotels. Together, they instilled in me a deep appreciation for whole foods and the dining experience. Between the frequent dinner parties they loved to host and the quality of food they chose to serve, they taught me that the best food involve basic techniques, fresh ingredients, and a whole lot of love.

While my interests have long gravitated toward natural healing modalities, integrative nutrition, and a holistic approach to wellness, I also spent many years working in the service industry, and my approach to food will always be as a passionate foodie, first and foremost. In fact, most people who know me would surely attest that I care passionately about what goes into my body yet refuse to eat food that simply isn't delicious.

It is with this simple philosophy in mind that I've written this book, taking care that each recipe is easy to make, healthful and nourishing, and always bursting with flavor.

In our busy, digitally driven lives, preparing and sharing a small, thoughtful bite that brings us back to something pure and tactile is a beautiful way to nourish both body and soul.

It is with much love in my heart that I present this collection of revitalizing, beautifying, and truly guilt-free plant-based recipes to help you celebrate your truest expression of beauty.

A WORD ABOUT YOUR SKIN

Although most of us would surely agree that our character and personality play a much more significant role in our overall attractiveness, our skin speaks volumes on our beauty as well. Physical glow is, after all, a direct reflection of our inner health. Yet very few of us truly take the time to recognize the control we actually have over our own physical, mental, and spiritual beauty. It is time to take back our glow.

The deepest, most profound change we can make to our health, beauty, and overall well-being starts in the kitchen. The foods we eat support our body's beautifying processes, breaking down into molecular building blocks and directly impacting the glow of our skin, the shine of our hair, and the radiance emanating from our very being.

The root of most illnesses is stagnation of the body's pathways and impaction of waste matter in its cells and tissues. Stagnation of the body's pathways creates a breeding ground for bacteria and viruses to thrive, triggering illness. Our skin is often the first place to show signs of this distress.

Processed, refined, and artificial foods are extremely difficult and often impossible for the body to break down, remaining in our system to occupy clean, healthy cells. Plants, on the other hand, absorb the powerful life force from the sun in the form of chlorophyll and bring that powerful energy into every cell in our body.

The foods we consume on a daily basis can either deplete us or invigorate us. Pack your diet with nature's most powerfully beautifying foods and deeply transform how you look and feel.

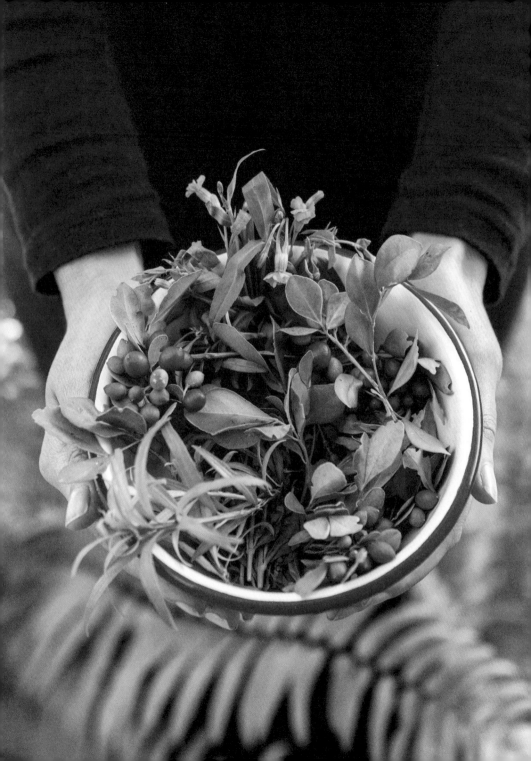

THE PRETTY ZEN PHILOSOPHY

The Pretty Zen philosophy is deeply rooted in finding, balancing, and maintaining wholesome beauty in a modern world. Part philosophy, part lifestyle, Pretty Zen takes natural healing modalities, Eastern philosophies, integrative nutrition, and an overall holistic approach to well-being and applies them to a modern way of life. It is a natural outlook with an underlying belief that there may be no greater pursuit than a life well loved.

The following beauty nutrition principles are at the core of the Pretty Zen philosophy and the beauty-boosting recipes in this book will help your body detox, repair, and prepare for your most radiant self.

ENZYMES: Enzymes are catalysts. On a physical level, enzymes help overcome digestive stagnation. They help with building raw materials, distributing nutrients, hormone balancing, and detoxification. On a spiritual level, they help fill you with vitality and overcome lethargy.

Enzyme-rich foods are activated and sprouted nuts and seeds, pineapple, papaya, mango, avocado, olive oils, and coconut oil.

RAW FOODS: Any whole food that has not been heated above 115°F has preserved its living enzymes and is considered raw. Enjoying an abundance of raw foods helps you load up on enzymes, minerals, and phytonutrients essential for restored digestion, increased energy, sharpened brain power, and glowing skin. That being said, raw foods can be difficult to digest if you are not in the habit of consuming them. Always pair raw vegetables with an abundance of healthy fats for easier digestion and nutrient absorption.

MINERALS: Everything we are physically made of, including our teeth, bones, skin, and internal organs, are composed of colloidal minerals, the living minerals found in plants. Eating an abundance of mineral-rich foods ensures that your body gets the collagen and connective tissue matter to nourish your skin, hair, and nails.

Cooked starchy foods containing high carbohydrates, such as bread, rice, pasta, white flour products, and refined sugar, run minerals out of the body and create blood sugar fluctuations. They also often lead to fungus, yeast, and mold overgrowth in the body.

ALKALINITY: The human body's ideal pH range is between 7.35 and 7.40, providing the optimal working environment for the body's fluids and tissues. Our blood pH is naturally alkaline.

Foods rich in alkaline minerals—calcium, magnesium, silicon, iron, sodium, and manganese—create alkalinity in the body and help magnetize waste matter out of the cells.

Foods rich in acidic minerals—phosphorous, chlorine, iodine, nitrogen, and sulfur—are also needed to be healthy and in balance; however, an excess of acidity throws our blood pH out of balance and can lead to inflammation, water retention, stiffness, and tissue degeneration.

AMINO ACIDS: Twenty percent of the human body is made up of protein. Proteins are large, complex molecules that are critical for the normal functioning of the human body. They are essential for the structure, function, and regulation of the body's tissues and organs. Proteins are made up of hundreds of smaller units called amino acids that are attached to one another by peptide bonds, forming a long chain.

The twenty amino acids that are found within proteins convey a vast array of chemical versatility. Humans can produce ten of the twenty amino acids. The others must be obtained in food on a daily basis because, unlike fat and starch, the human body does not store excess amino acids for later use.

It's a common misconception that animal protein is superior to the protein found in plant foods. Plant-based foods are a source of all amino acids and are easier for the body to digest. It is also not necessary to combine plant proteins at each meal to form complete proteins. Your body can do that on its own.

HEALTHY FATS: Sixty percent of the brain is made of fat. We need good fat for healthy brain function, hormone production, to strengthen cell membranes, and to keep the intestines and joints lubricated. Fat is best derived from such foods as avocados, olives, raw or cold-pressed olive oil, seed oils, nuts, seeds, and young coconuts.

PREBIOTICS AND PROBIOTICS: Our gut accounts for two-thirds of our immune system. Gut bacteria influence digestion, allergies, and metabolism. It can also affect our mental health and sleep, and shed light on the cravings we have for certain foods.

A primal connection exists between our brain and our gut. We often talk about a "gut feeling" or "trusting our gut instinct." This mind-gut connection is more than metaphorical. Our brain and gut are connected by an extensive network of neurons and a highway of chemicals and hormones that provide continual feedback on our state of hunger, our stress levels, and possible disease-causing microbes entering our body. Making sure to eat nondigestible fibrous foods, known as prebiotics—such as bananas, dandelion greens, onion, and garlic—which feed on the good bacteria we already have in our system, and probiotics—such as fermented foods, kombucha, nut milks, and cheeses—that help increase the healthy flora in our system, help our gut function at its best and our skin glowing.

ADAPTOGENS: Our ability to recover from the effects of stress decreases as we age. The stress hormone cortisol tends to linger for longer periods of time, damaging the skin's collagen and natural moisture levels. Adrenaline also increases during stress, decreasing blood flow, diverting oxygen away from skin, and allowing for toxin build up.

Adaptogens are a unique class of healing plants that help balance, restore, and protect the body and its physiological functions. Adding adaptogens, such as Cordycep mushroom, astragalus root, rhodiola, ashwaganda, and holy basil, to your routine can make you more resilient to the damaging effects of stress levels.

FOOD COMBINING

You can be eating the purest foods, but if you don't adhere to basic food-combining principles, you may be creating arduous work for your digestive system. Ill-combined foods can create carbonic gas, a noxious by-product of food sitting on old matter in the body, which causes inflammation, bone decalcification, and body odor.

Follow these steps to reduce the digestive load and to free up energy for health and beauty:

BASIC FOOD COMBINING GUIDELINES

- Starches with starches
- Protein with protein
- Any combination of nuts, seeds, dried fruits, and bananas
- Fresh fruits alone and on an empty stomach
- Raw vegetables paired with all meals
- Cooked vegetables with starches and cooked nonstarch vegetables with proteins

MINDFUL EATING

SAVOR YOUR MEALS: Taking the time to savor and enjoy our meals is one of the healthiest things we can do. We are more likely to chew our food more, notice sooner when we are full, and even notice flavors we might otherwise have missed.

Mindfulness is also about rekindling a relationship with food and connecting with the story behind our meals. When we pause to consider all of the people involved in the preparation of our meal, from the loved ones who prepared it, to those who planted and harvested the raw ingredients, to the water, soil, and other elements that were part of its creation, it is hard not to feel both grateful and interconnected. We not only gain a deeper appreciation for our nutrition, but our shopping habits might change in the process, too.

EATING WITH THE SEASONS: Building a lifestyle around seasonal food facilitates the body's natural healing process.

Springtime foods are detoxifying; summertime foods are light and cooling; fall foods are grounding; and wintertime foods are heavy and warming. Choosing local, seasonal ingredients will help support our overall well-being.

PRIMARY FOOD: Primary food is the concept that our need for relationships, connection, love, movement, happiness, pleasure, spirituality, purpose, and fulfillment satisfies our hunger for life.

When primary food is in balance and being regularly nourished, what we eat is secondary in our mind.

CONSCIOUS EATING: Our mind and body are deeply interconnected. Taking the time to slow down and really chew our food properly can make a world of difference to the digestion process. Strive to chew each mouthful of your food thirty times. The act of slowing down while eating will heighten your pleasure and your connection to yourself and others.

Everyone's body is multidimensional and unique. The most valuable beauty skills you'll ever learn are listening to your unique body and understanding how it responds to different forms of nourishment. The Pretty Zen philosophy encompasses more than just food and nutrition. Stress management, exercise, healthy and supportive relationships, restful sleep, hydration, and tending to our spiritual, mental, and physical happiness are crucial components to our overall beauty and I touch more on those topics in my Pretty Zen sister book: *Fresh & Pure: Organically Crafted Beauty Balms & Cleansers.*

Beauty Kitchen Tips

- *As much as possible, eat foods without a label or packaging, but at the very least, make sure you can recognize and pronounce every ingredient on the label.*

- *Support local food, farmers, and artisans as much as possible. Always opt for whole foods, organic when possible, that you can trace back to its source. Remember, we all vote with our dollar.*

- *If you consume animal products, make sure you can trace your food back to the source and know where the animal has been raised and fed. The well-being of the animal you consume matters for your own health and for the environment. Make sure that it has been humanely raised.*

- *Avoid the "whites": white bread, pasta, rice, refined sugar, high-fructose sweeteners, trans fats, and canned foods that are not free of bisphenol-A (BPA).*

- *Spend more time enjoying food, sharing it with people you love, and freeing yourself from calorie counting, restrictive diets, and nutritional dogmas.*

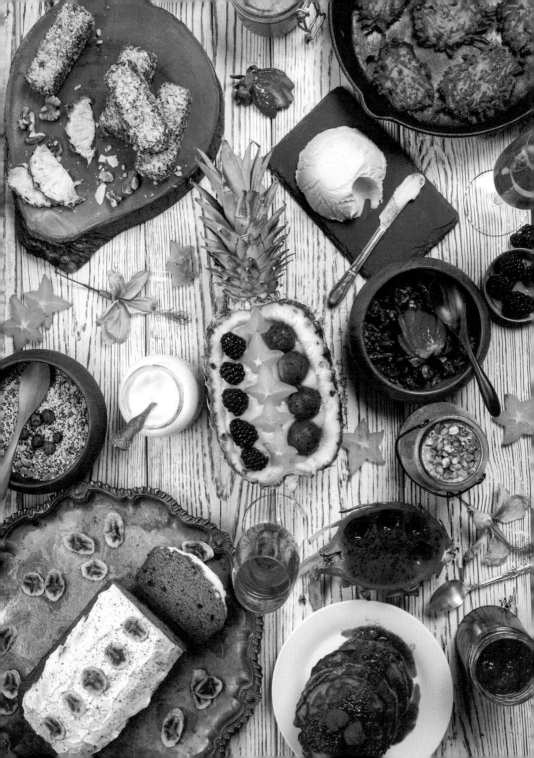

THE BEAUTY KITCHEN

PANTRY PRIMERS

Let's help you stock a powerful beauty kitchen. Armed with a well-stocked pantry and a few simple cooking techniques, you can prepare many new and exciting, healthful meals.

You may need to upgrade your pantry with a few new ingredients initially, yet once your kitchen is stocked with the following beauty foods, you'll never be more than minutes away from a quick, deliciously nourishing meal.

BEAUTY-BOOSTING FOODS

AVOCADOS: Antioxidant-rich avocados are rich in vitamin E, which keeps skin cells healthy and strong, and B vitamins responsible for DNA repair. Avocados are also one of the healthiest sources of fat and can help reduce "bad" cholesterol levels.

BEETS: This humble root vegetable holds a wealth of nutrients, including beta-carotene, folic acid, fiber, and iron. The leafy greens are even more nutritious, with double the potassium, folic acid, calcium, and iron.

BERRIES: Almost all berries rank among the world's most nutritious fruits. Their concentrated micronutrients make them one of the best sources of antioxidants for glowing skin.

BLACK RICE: A naturally gluten-free grain, black rice is high in protein, dietary fiber, and anti-inflammatory properties, and has one of the highest levels of anthocyanin antioxidants of any food. It is also a good source of iron.

BUCKWHEAT: Nutty, savory buckwheat, despite its name, does not contain wheat or gluten. It's a nutritious alternative to white flour, with high levels of iron, magnesium, protein, and fiber.

CACAO: A prized food of the Maya, cacao is the raw, natural source of one of the most cherished treats of all time: chocolate! And in its unprocessed form, cacao ranks as one of the most antioxidant-rich foods in the world. Cacao is also a good source of minerals and is one of the top plant-based sources of magnesium.

CHIA SEEDS: A staple food for the Aztecs and Maya, chia, which in ancient Mayan meant "strength," was a prized food that helped provide sustainable energy. The tiny seed is loaded with fiber, protein, omega-3 fatty acids, and a variety of micronutrients.

CITRUS (LEMONS, LIMES, ORANGES, AND SO ON): Keeps the body alkaline, helps boost immunity and circulation, and fights inflammation.

When peeling citrus fruits, leave on the white pith, full of fiber-rich pectin, which helps absorb plant-based iron. And don't toss the peel if it's organic; the outermost layer, the zest, offers limonoids, a bitter-tasting lipid that protects the fruit from fungi and is a powerful anticarcinogen.

COCONUT OIL: Extracted from the flesh of the coconut, coconut oil is similar to dairy butter without the cholesterol. Made of medium-chain fatty acids that quickly assimilate in the body for instant energy, this saturated fat is essential for healthy cell membranes. You can find coconut oil in the natural section of most grocery stores.

DATES: Contain selenium, manganese, copper, and magnesium, all of which are integral to healthy bone development and strength. They are also a great source of fiber, iron, vitamin A, and many B vitamins as well. They provide an instant energy boost and are one of the best sources for potassium. Use them as a sweetener in your smoothies and baked goods.

FRUITS AND VEGETABLES: The only rules when it comes to fruits and veggies are: eat a wide variety, eat as organic as possible, and eat as many as possible. For the small amount of calories they contain, they deliver the most nutrients of any class of food. Vegetables are an excellent low-calorie source of vitamins, minerals, and fiber for healthy cell repair and for strong, beautiful glowing hair, nails, and skin.

GOJI BERRIES: Also called wolfberries, or "red diamonds" due to their unusually high nutritional value, these fruits are native to southeastern Europe and Asia. They are characterized by their bright orange-red color and raisinlike shape. They have been cultivated in Asia for more than two thousand years, where Traditional Chinese Medicine has been using the berries for medicinal purposes. They are an excellent source of antioxidants, such as polyphenols, flavonoids, and carotenoids, and vitamins A, C, and E.

GREEN LEAFY VEGETABLES: Exceptionally high in chlorophyll, these greens oxygenate your blood and boost your body's production of antiaging nutrients due to their vitamins, minerals, protein, fiber, and a rich dose of collagen-building vitamin C.

HEMP SEEDS: Shelled hemp seeds are a complete source of protein that support healthy cell building and repair. They are also an excellent source of omega fatty acids, including gamma-lineolenic acid, a rich source for beautiful glowing skin, hair, and nails.

MACA ROOT POWDER: A member of the cruciferous family, maca root powder has been consumed for its medicinal benefits for thousands of years in regions of the Andes Mountains. Considered an "adaptogen," maca helps the body naturally adapt to stressors, and also has a positive effect on hormone balance, energy levels, and stamina.

MAQUI BERRY POWDER: One of the highest-known antioxidant fruits in the world, the maqui berry has a strong concentration of polyphenols and anthocyanins, which repair and protect DNA and improve brain function. Fresh maqui berries are not available in North America but a freeze-dried powder can be found online and in health food stores.

MATCHA: A finely ground powder of a specific green tea that is shade-grown for about three weeks before harvest, producing more chlorophyll, heanine, and caffeine. Matcha is known to induce a calm energy. The antioxidant-rich tea helps support skin health by reducing inflammation and free radicals that accelerate skin aging.

MUSHROOMS: Of all the earth's natural substances, mushrooms are among the most medicinal. They enhance the immune system and fight free radicals.

NUTRITIONAL YEAST: Affectionately known as "nooch," this is an inactive form of yeast that has a cheesy, nutty flavor. It is often used as a vegan cheese sprinkle and can add an invaluable cheesy flavor to dishes. Rich in protein, minerals, and especially B vitamins, it makes a great nutritional supplement. Nooch can be found in most natural food stores or from online food retailers.

NUTS AND SEEDS: Nuts and seeds are extremely high in life-sustaining nutrients, including healthy fats, minerals, protein, and fiber.

OLIVE OIL: Loaded with vitamin E, olive oil strengthens cell membranes and works with vitamin C to keep skin looking youthful. It is an antioxidant-rich oil that is known to reduce the risk of heart disease and high blood pressure.

QUINOA: A complete protein with nine of the essential amino acids, quinoa is a gluten-free seed packed with trace minerals such as iron, zinc, and magnesium. A low-glycemic complex carbohydrate, quinoa keeps blood sugar balanced while supporting healthy digestion.

RAW APPLE CIDER VINEGAR: This light, golden brown vinegar is made from organic, unpasteurized apple cider. Look for raw apple cider vinegar that contains the edible sediment known as the "mother."

SEA VEGETABLES: Packed with omega-3s, protein, and beauty minerals that feed your skin, hair, and nails, sea plants—such as kelp, kombu, dulse, wakame, and spirulina—are veritable superfoods. Add flakes to salads, cook in broths and nourish bowls, or add powders to smoothies or nut milks.

SPROUTS: Condensed nutrition at its finest and easy to grow right on your kitchen countertop, sprouts are incredibly rich in enzymes, vitamins, minerals, chlorophyll, antioxidants, and even protein.

SWEETENERS: Replace all refined sugars, including cane sugar, cane juice, fructose, and corn syrup, with healthier alternatives, such as stevia, dates, Grade B pure maple syrup, coconut sugar, raw honey, yacon, and unsulfured blackstrap molasses. These natural alternatives have a lower glycemic index and have health benefits when used in moderation.

TAHINI: This thick paste, made of sesame seeds, adds a creamy, nutty, earthy flavor to dishes. Rich in minerals, omega fatty acids, and B vitamins, tahini is available in the natural section of most grocery stores.

TAMARI/COCONUT AMINOS: Tamari is a gluten-free version of soy sauce; for a soy-free version, use coconut aminos. You can find tamari and coconut aminos in most health food stores and online food retailers.

EAT THE RAINBOW

The easiest way to ensure you have a varied diet is to incorporate fruits and vegetables in a broad spectrum of colors. Each hue is nature's color code to certain nutrients that help your body function at its best. Here's the breakdown:

RED: Several compounds give red-hued produce their color: flavonoids and carotenoids (including lycopene). These antioxidants help destroy free radicals in the body and may help with heart health and graceful aging. Sources: tomatoes, watermelon, cherries, strawberries, red peppers, red cabbage.

ORANGE: Orange-hued produce is rich in beta-carotene, a powerful antioxidant, which the body converts into vitamin A and often vitamin C. These nutrients support a host of body functions to help immune function and healthy skin. Sources: butternut squash, oranges, carrots, mangoes, pumpkins, sweet potato, pineapple, cantaloupe.

YELLOW: The yellow in produce comes from the carotenoid zeaxanthin and beta-cryptoxanthin, powerful vitamin antioxidants, vital for healthy cell growth, bone and skin health, and immunity. Sources: corn, papayas, yellow bell peppers, lemons, yellow grapefruit.

GREEN: Green produce is particularly rich in folate (folic acid), which plays an important role in cell division, makes red blood cells, and supplies lutein, vital for eye health. Sources: collard greens, kale, Brussels sprouts, spinach, lettuces.

BLUE, INDIGO, AND VIOLET: Anthocyanins are responsible for those vivid blue and black colors in produce. These support healthy aging and cardiovascular disease biomarkers. Because concentrations of anthocyanins vary among fruits and vegetables, eat a variety as part of your nutritious diet to reap the most benefits. Sources: plums or prunes, purple grapes, red cabbage, blueberries, blackberries.

GLOW-GETTING HERBS AND SPICES

Basil: Antiaging, anti-inflammatory

Black peppercorns: Aid in nutrient absorption, increase metabolism

Cardamom: Promotes heart health, aids digestion

Cayenne pepper: Reduces inflammation, boosts metabolism

Chili powder: Regulates blood pressure, reduces pain

Cilantro: Soothes sore throat, speeds digestion

Cinnamon: Helps control blood sugar, reduces bad cholesterol

Dill: Helps control levels of blood cholesterol, a natural antioxidant

Ginger: Aids digestion, soothes upset stomach, anti-inflammatory

Garlic: Protects against heart disease, antibacterial, antiviral

Mustard: Improves circulation, relieves congestion

Oregano: Antibacterial, antifungal, reduces inflammation

Parsley: Calms nerves, natural antioxidant

Rosemary: Improves digestion, enhances concentration

Sea salt: Offers trace minerals that have been processed out of table salt

Thyme: Reduces inflammation, controls blood pressure

Turmeric: Regulates hormones, boosts metabolism, anti-inflammatory

Wasabi: Improves circulation, boosts metabolism

When to Insist on Organic

The Environmental Working Group (ewg.org), a nonprofit that aims to protect public health and the environment, has determined that we can reduce the amount of pesticides we ingest by 90 percent by choosing to buy the organic versions of the following twelve fruits and veggies, it calls the Dirty Dozen: apples, celery, cherries, grapes, lettuce, nectarines, peaches, pears, potatoes, spinach, strawberries, and sweet bell peppers.

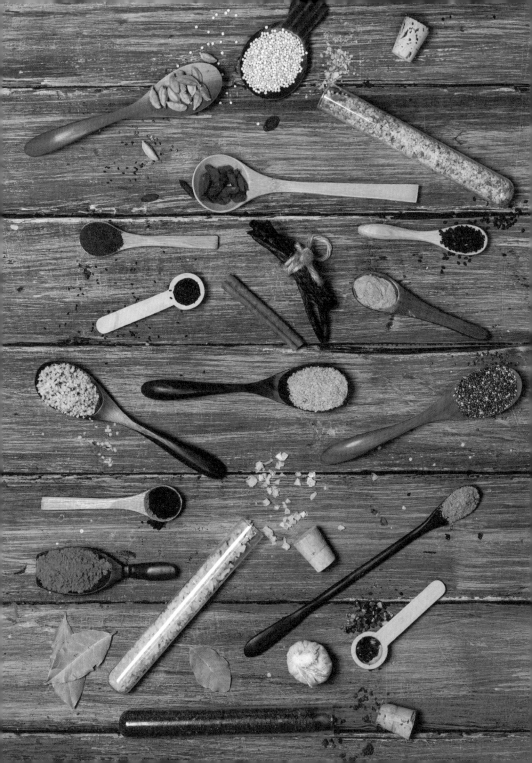

KITCHEN TOOL ESSENTIALS

To make the most of the recipes in this book, you'll only need a few essential tools. These key tools will help you save time and make food prep more efficient and more enjoyable:

CERAMIC NONSTICK PAN: A convenient cooking surface that prevents food from sticking while cooking. Most, however, contain extremely toxic chemicals. Look for Eco Pans. These ceramic pans use eco-friendly substances to produce a nonstick surface for easier, nontoxic cooking.

FOOD PROCESSOR: Food processors excel at chopping, grating, and shredding, perfect for making salsas and hummus and for slicing veggies for slaw.

DEHYDRATOR: A dehydrator is an ovenlike appliance that uses low temperatures and a fan to dry food. It essentially removes the moisture from food, while keeping the enzymes of your raw food intact. Although you can prepare every recipe in this book without one, a dehydrator is a fun, useful machine for making everything from fruit leathers and jerky to crackers and crisps.

GLASS JARS WITH LIDS/AIRTIGHT CONTAINERS: They make perfect storage containers for the pantry and the fridge, are safe for hot foods and liquids, are reusable, and don't pose harmful risks to environmental or personal health. Try to avoid plastic containers as much as possible. Ceramic, stoneware, or stainless-steel containers are great choices, too.

HIGH-SPEED BLENDER: Blenders are the best tool for liquefying ingredients, perfect for smoothies, pureed soups, and sauces. High-performance blenders will also grind nuts to make milks, cheeses, and nut butters.

MANDOLINE: Although not essential to have, a mandoline is a useful vegetable slicer that creates uniform slices, such as vegetables for salads and chips, as well as some specialty cuts, such as waffle-cut and matchsticks for fries. The plastic version of the more costly, stainless-steel model is actually easier to use, clean, and store and is extremely handy to have around.

SPIRALIZER: Spiral vegetable slicers or spiralizers are kitchen appliances used for cutting vegetables—such as zucchini, potatoes, cucumbers, carrots, apples, and beets—into spaghetti-like strands that can be used as an alternative to pasta.

Know the Code

On the bottom of plastic food storage containers, you'll find a tiny triangle with a number (resin identification code), ranging from 1 to 7, inside, indicating the type of plastic. In general, the safest choices for food use are numbers 1, 2, 4, and 5. That's because number 3 is vinyl or polyvinyl chloride (PVC), 6 is polystyrene, and 7 can be various plastics. Some plastic containers with the resin codes of 3 and 7 may contain bisphenol-A (BPA).

A NOTE ABOUT THE RECIPES

The following recipes have been created with the most naturally nourishing ingredients for your body. They are versatile and flexible, no matter what your dietary preferences are.

All the recipes in this book are dairy-free, gluten-free, refined-sugar-free, and plant-based.

A note about buckwheat, amaranth, teff, wild rice, and quinoa: Although technically seeds, these pseudo-cereals, or super seeds as they are called, have many of the same properties as grain. They do not contain gluten and are easier to digest, high in protein, and rich sources of complex carbohydrates.

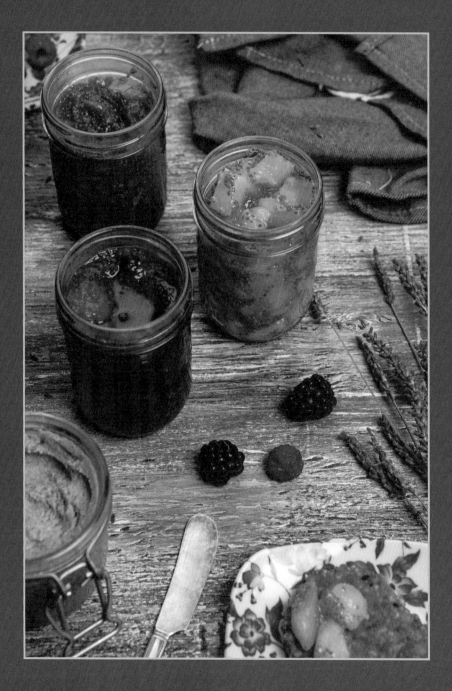

MORNING STARTERS

Dishes Worth Getting Out of Bed For

Literally meaning "breaking the fast," your morning starters should be chosen carefully as to not overburden your system after a night of rest and fasting. Taking it slow and easy and choosing nutrient-dense breakfast items with a healthy dose of protein and healthy fats and that are low in sugar will help set the tone for an energy-fueled day full of beauty potential. The following recipes are simple, energizing meals you can enjoy every day, with a few, slower, lingering weekend brunch items.

How to Build a Smoothie Bowl

Smoothie bowls are the perfect excuse to have dessert for breakfast. Here are a few tricks to achieve the right consistency, proportions, and most important, nutrition.

- **KEEP IT THICK.** Start with less liquid than you normally would for a drinkable smoothie, or add extra base ingredients, such as frozen fruit or veggies, to the blender. The fruit foundation makes added sugars unnecessary, so you'll get naturally sweet fuel for the rest of your day.

- **KEEP IT COOL.** Have all your topping ingredients prepped and ready to go. Chilling your bowl before getting started is also a great idea.

- **KEEP IT TEXTURED.** What really makes a smoothie bowl different from its drinkable counterpart are the toppings.

For a balance of flavors and textures, choose at least one topping from each of the categories below:

- **THE FRUIT:** Fresh seasonal fruit is best; choose a mix of berries, citrus, and tropical varieties.

- **THE CRUNCH:** Choose from toasted coconut flakes, nuts, seeds, cacao nibs, or granola.

- **THE HEALTH-BOOSTERS:** To keep your macronutrients balanced, add almond milk or a nut butter to get your proteins and fats. Try chia seeds, hemp seeds, or goji berries for an extra punch of nutrients.

- **THE SWEETENER:** A drizzle of pure maple syrup, only if needed.

RAW CHOCOLATE ACAI BOWL

The original smoothie bowl, made with the acai berry, is a traditional dish eaten on the beaches of Brazil. Dubbed the "Beauty Berry" by Brazilians, acai berries are small, dark purple berries that truly pack a whole host of antioxidants, amino acids, and essential fatty acids. It's a delicious way to protect the skin from environmental aggressors and to reduce the appearance of aging.

SERVES 1 TO 2

1 to 2 frozen bananas
2 tablespoons acai powder
1 tablespoon raw cacao powder
½ cup strawberries, hulled
1 cup almond milk
2 tablespoons cacao nibs (optional)

Combine all the ingredients in a blender and blend to a thick, smooth consistency. Spoon into a bowl and top with seasonal berries or try with the Chocolate Cherry Goji Grain-Free Granola (page 37).

✦ ✦ ✦ ✦

KITCHEN NOTE

Freezing bananas are an excellent way to save bananas that are past their prime. Frozen bananas also provide the perfect ice-creamy texture for smoothies and smoothie bowls. Just peel, slice, and store in your freezer until ready to use.

✦ ✦ ✦ ✦

SUPERSEED MUESLI WITH BLISSFULL BLUE MYLK

Instead of grains or oats, this muesli cereal contains some of my favorite seeds, all rich in fiber, complex carbohydrates, protein, minerals, and skin-beautifying omega-3 fatty acids for instantly usable fuel that will rev up your energy for the day. Best of all, it's perfectly customizable. Here you'll find a raw and a cooked version. Try them both and decide your favorite.

SUPERSEED MUESLI

MAKES 6 CUPS

2 cups buckwheat groats

1 cup hemp seeds

1 cup millet

1 cup uncooked quinoa

½ cup sesame seeds

½ cup sunflower seeds

1 tablespoon ground cinnamon

BLISSFUL BLUE MYLK

MAKES 2 CUPS

2 cups almond milk

½ teaspoon spirulina powder

¼ cup blueberries

To make the muesli:
Place all the muesli ingredients in a large bowl and stir. Store in an airtight container at room temperature for up to 3 months.

To make the mylk:
Combine all the mylk ingredients in a blender and process until smooth. Store in an airtight bottle in the refrigerator for 2 to 3 days.

To prepare raw:
Combine ½ cup of the muesli and 1 cup of mylk in a bowl. Allow to soak for 20 minutes. Top with your desired garnish.

To prepare cooked:
Bring 1 cup of water to a boil in a medium saucepan. Add ½ cup of the muesli and cook over low heat for 15 minutes, or until the water has almost evaporated. Remove from the heat and pour in 1 cup mylk. Cover and let sit for an additional 5 minutes.

+ + + +

KITCHEN NOTE

Divide the muesli among mason jars and top with fruit for an easy, on-the-go treat.

+ + + +

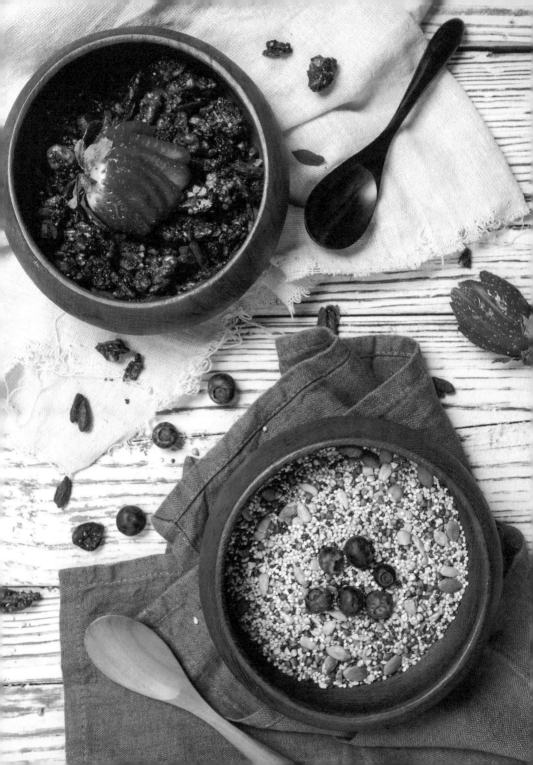

CHOCOLATE CHERRY GOJI GRAIN-FREE GRANOLA

Finally! You can have chocolate for breakfast! This deliciously satisfying chocolaty treat packs a serious crunch and punch in the way of healthy fats, omega-3s, and protein from the various nuts and seeds. Raw cacao, the purest form of chocolate, supports skin with a concentrated dose of antioxidants that block free radicals, protecting blood flow to the skin to keep it healthy and glowing.

MAKES 8 CUPS

2 cups slivered raw almonds

2 cups raw pecans

1 cup raw walnuts

1 cup pumpkin seeds

3 tablespoons chia seeds

1 teaspoon ground cardamom

¼ cup raw cacao powder

¼ teaspoon sea salt

1 tablespoon pure vanilla extract

¼ cup coconut oil

¼ cup pure maple syrup

½ cup Medjool dates, pitted and chopped

½ cup dried cherries

¼ cup goji berries

(continued)

2 tablespoons coconut flakes
2 tablespoons sunflower seeds
2 tablespoons cacao nibs
2 tablespoons hemp seeds
2 tablespoons flaxseed meal

Preheat the oven to 350°F. Line a baking sheet with parchment paper.

Combine the nuts, seeds, cardamom, cacao powder, and salt in a large bowl.

Place the coconut oil, maple syrup, and vanilla in a small saucepan over low heat, heat until warm, pour over the nut mixture, and mix well.

Spread the mixture evenly on the prepared baking sheet and bake for 20 minutes. Remove from the oven, add the dried cherries, dates, goji berries, and your desired add-ins, and stir.

Return the pan to the oven for another 10 minutes.

Once the granola is visibly browned, remove from the oven and let cool completely.

Store in an airtight glass container in a cool, dry place. For maximum freshness, use within 2 weeks.

✦ ✦ ✦ ✦

KITCHEN NOTE

This is a versatile granola recipe that works with an assortment of nuts, seeds, and dried fruit and I encourage you to create your own personalized variation!

✦ ✦ ✦ ✦

BLACK RICE PUDDING WITH COCONUT-MANGO CREAM

A traditional Balinese breakfast, black rice pudding is a wonderfully sweet, grounding dish that can also be enjoyed as a satisfying dessert. Although the pudding can be topped with any of your favorite seasonal fruits, it's exceptionally well paired with the sumptuous coconut-mango topping.

SERVES 2 TO 4

RICE PUDDING

2 cups coconut water

1 cup uncooked black rice

1 tablespoon coconut sugar

2 teaspoons pure vanilla extract

1 cup canned pure coconut milk

COCONUT-MANGO CREAM

1 ripe mango, peeled, pitted, and sliced

2 tablespoons coconut cream (see directions)

Coconut flakes

To make the rice pudding:

Combine the coconut water, rice, coconut sugar, and vanilla in a saucepan over medium heat and bring to a boil. Lower the heat and simmer, uncovered, stirring occasionally for 30 minutes, until the rice is tender.

Spoon out the thick top layer of coconut cream from the coconut milk can and set aside in a bowl. Empty the rest of the can of coconut milk into the

(continued)

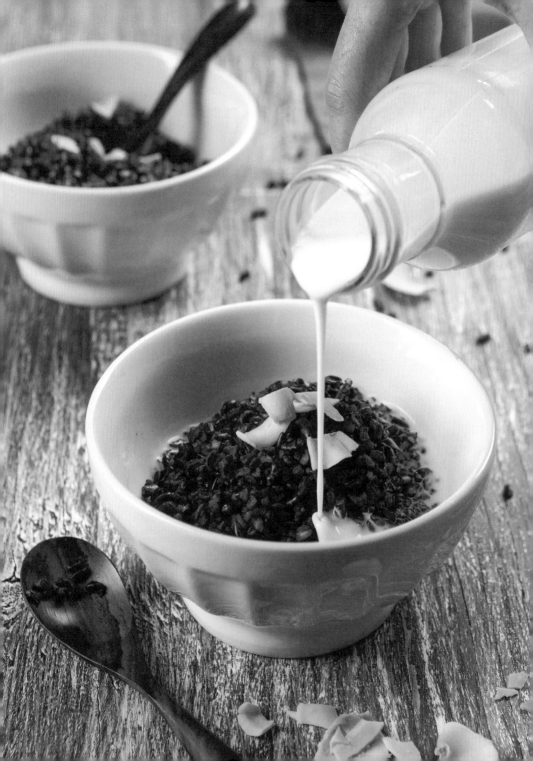

pudding mixture and bring to a simmer. Cook for another 5 minutes, stirring occasionally, until the mixture is creamy. Remove from the heat.

To make the coconut-mango cream:
Place the reserved coconut cream and the mango slices in a blender and blend.

Meanwhile, toast the coconut flakes in a small, dry pan over medium heat for 3 minutes, until golden and fragrant.

To serve, spoon the pudding into bowls and top with a dollop of coconut-mango cream and a sprinkle of toasted coconut flakes.

✦　✦　✦　✦

BEAUTY FOOD SPOTLIGHT

Black rice contains anthocyanins, the same plant pigments responsible for the health benefits of other colorful plant foods, including maqui berries, blackberries, tart cherries, and beets. Anthocyanins help repair damaged cells and promote the growth of strong healthy hair and nails. They also contain powerful anti-inflammatory agents that help you manage weight and keep bloat away.

✦　✦　✦　✦

BANANA BREAD

This perfectly moist banana bread, bursting with flavor is a nourishing breakfast option with a macronutrient balance of fiber, protein, carbohydrates, and healthful fats that regulate your blood sugar and, in turn, support beautifully healthy skin aging.

MAKES 1 LOAF, 10 TO 12 SLICES

¼ cup melted coconut oil, plus more for pan

4 bananas

¼ cup pure maple syrup

2 teaspoons pure vanilla extract

1½ cups certified gluten-free oat flour

¾ cup almond meal

1 teaspoon baking powder

½ teaspoon baking soda

¼ teaspoon salt

Preheat the oven to 350°F. Grease an 8-inch loaf pan with coconut oil and set aside.

Combine the bananas, coconut oil, maple syrup, and vanilla in a blender and blend.

Transfer to a medium bowl and add the oat flour, almond meal, baking powder, baking soda, and salt. Whisk together and pour the batter evenly into the prepared pan. Bake for 60 to 70 minutes, or until a toothpick inserted into the center comes out clean.

Allow to cool before enjoying.

KITCHEN NOTE

As a special treat, serve with a generous topping of maple-glazed toasted walnuts.

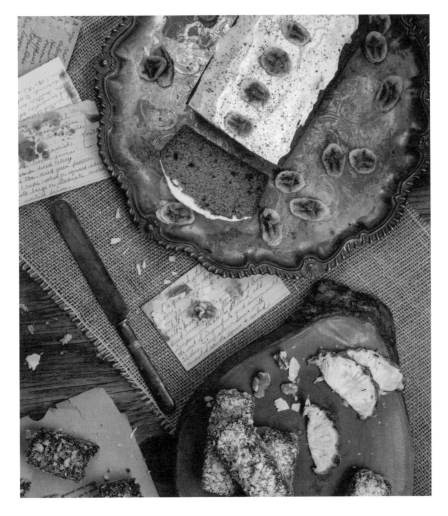

RAW PIÑA COLADA BREAKFAST BARS

Pineapple and coconut are a match made in heaven, and now the tropical combo can get you out of bed with the promise of gorgeous skin. These wholesome, raw bars packed with antioxidants protect the body from free radical damage, keeping the skin blemish free.

MAKES 10 TO 12 BARS

½ cup dried figs
½ cup raw almonds
½ cup raw cashews
1 cup raw pecans
½ cup raw pumpkin seeds
½ cup raw sunflower seeds
½ cup unsweetened dried pineapple chunks
1 teaspoon pure vanilla extract
½ cup dried shredded coconut

Soak the figs in a bowl of water for 1 hour. Drain, chop, and set aside.

Combine the nuts and seeds in a food processor and process until chunky. Add the figs, pineapple, and vanilla and process until the mixture begins to stick together. Add the coconut and process briefly to incorporate, leaving the dough chunky for texture. Check the consistency of your dough. If your dough is too wet, add a few nuts and process. If the dough isn't sticky enough, add 1 teaspoon of water at a time, until you obtain a sticky, moldable dough.

Place the dough on a large sheet of plastic wrap and wrap it tightly. Using a rolling pin, roll the dough into a large rectangle about ½ inch thick. Unwrap and slice into bars or bites as preferred. Store in an airtight container in the refrigerator for 2 weeks.

SWEET POTATO LATKES WITH ZA'ATAR YOGURT

If you love a good latke, you'll love this sweet, earthy twist on the classic crispy potato pancake. Made with the healthier sweet potato, added carrots, and warm spices, this lighter, brighter panfried variety will leave you nourished and satisfied. A scoop of za'atar yogurt makes a spicy-cool garnish.

MAKES 8 TO 12

ZA'ATAR YOGURT
1 cup Coconut Yogurt (page 202)
1 teaspoon Za'atar (page 208)

LATKES
2 tablespoons flaxseed meal
6 tablespoons warm water
2 cups shredded sweet potato (medium grate)
1 cup shredded carrot (medium grate)
½ cup diced white onion
½ teaspoon grated fresh or ground turmeric
1 teaspoon ground cumin
Sea salt and freshly ground black pepper
¼ cup coconut oil

To make the za'atar yogurt:
Place the yogurt in a bowl, stir in the za'atar, and place in the refrigerator to chill.

(continued)

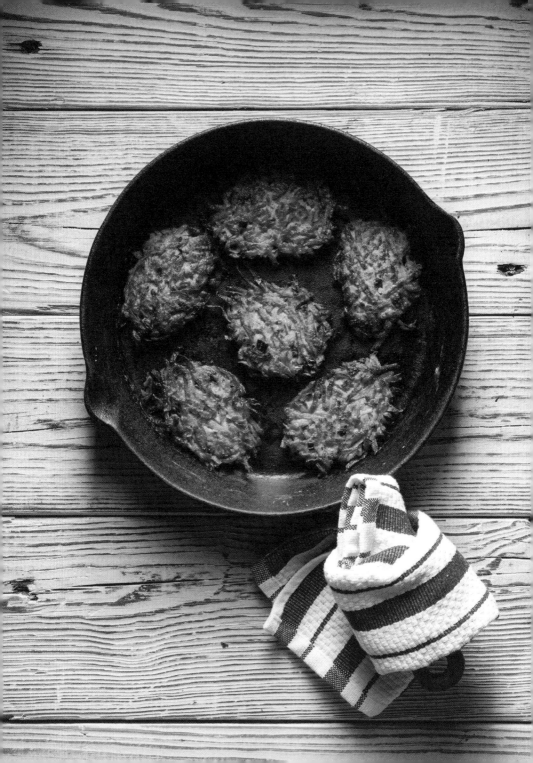

To make the latkes:

Prepare two flax eggs by combining the warm water with the flaxseed meal in a small bowl. Stir and let sit for 10 minutes.

Place the shredded sweet potato and carrot in large bowl. Drain the vegetables of any excess liquid and stir in the flax eggs, onion, turmeric, cumin, and salt and pepper to taste.

Heat 1 tablespoon of the coconut oil in a large skillet over medium heat. Press a heaping tablespoon of the mixture onto the skillet. Working in batches, cook the latkes until golden brown, 4 to 5 minutes per side, adding the remaining oil by the tablespoon between batches. Line a plate with a paper towel and place the cooked latkes on it to drain any excess oil. Transfer to a serving platter.

To serve, top each latke with a dollop of za'atar yogurt.

✦   ✦   ✦   ✦

BEAUTY FOOD SPOTLIGHT

The high content of beta-carotene in sweet potatoes, which helps convert vitamin A in your body, is also responsible for producing new skin cells, greatly enhancing the glow of your skin.

✦   ✦   ✦   ✦

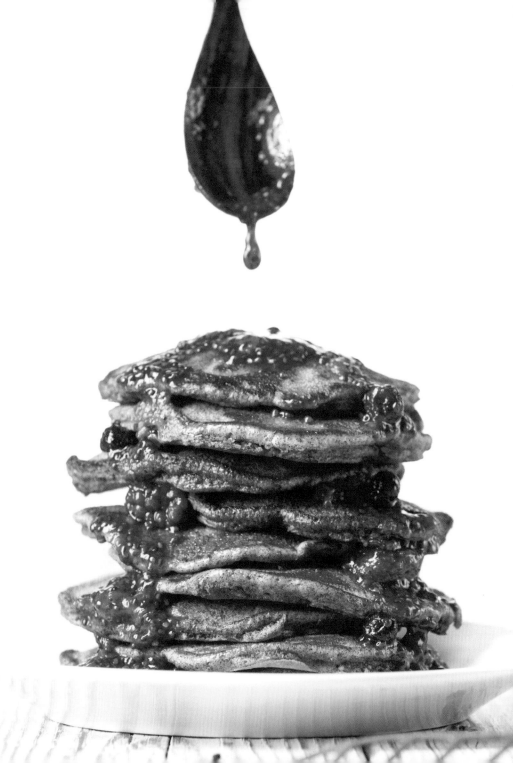

BUCKWHEAT PANCAKES WITH MIXED BERRY COMPOTE

Despite its name, buckwheat contains no wheat. In fact, it is technically a seed—a nutrient-packed, gluten-free seed high in both protein and fiber.

These delicious, nutritious pancakes are low on the glycemic index and high in the phytochemical rutin, a special beauty nutrient that has regenerative antiaging properties. Rutin also strengthens blood vessels, which can prevent varicose veins.

SERVES 2 TO 4

PANCAKES

1 cup almond milk

2 tablespoons raw apple cider vinegar

½ cup buckwheat flour

½ cup certified gluten-free oat flour

1 teaspoon baking powder

¼ teaspoon baking soda

½ teaspoon sea salt

1 banana, mashed

1 teaspoon pure vanilla extract

1 tablespoon coconut oil, plus more for grilling

2 tablespoons pure maple syrup

(continued)

1 cup mixed berries
¼ cup water
1 tablespoon pure maple syrup
1 tablespoon fresh lemon juice

To make the pancakes:

Mix the almond milk and vinegar together in a bowl and let sit for 5 minutes.

Stir the flours, baking powder, baking soda, and salt together in a medium bowl. Add the banana, vanilla, coconut oil, and maple syrup as well as the vinegar mixture and stir together until fully blended. For best texture and flavor, let the batter sit for 15 minutes.

Lightly oil the bottom of a nonstick skillet with coconut oil and heat over medium heat. When the oil is hot, pour ⅓ to ½ cup of batter into the skillet. Cook until small bubbles form in the middle, 3 to 4 minutes. Flip and cook for about 2 minutes more on the opposite side. Repeat until all the batter is used, adding oil to the skillet as needed between pancakes.

To make the compote:

Combine all the compote ingredients in a saucepan and bring to a simmer over medium-low heat, stirring to dissolve the syrup. Simmer for another minute, until the berries have softened. Remove from the heat and let cool.

Serve the pancakes topped with a generous dollop of berry compote.

UPGRADE YOUR PB AND J

Ah, the peanut butter and jelly sandwich, a comforting classic that hardly needs improving in the taste department. With just a few easy upgrades, you can easily boost the nutritional game of this favorite childhood staple.

SUPERSEED BUTTER

Swap out the peanuts for skin-nourishing almonds and cashews and give your nut butter a serious nutritional boost from the hemp seeds, sunflower seeds, chia seeds, and maca powder. Not only will you benefit from the hormone-balancing, free-radical-neutralizing, and beautifying essential amino acids, protein, fiber, and healthy fats, but you'll also enjoy a sticky, satisfying, nutty spread.

MAKES 2 CUPS

1 cup raw almonds
1 cup raw cashews
½ cup raw sunflower seeds
½ cup raw hemp seeds
1 tablespoon chia seeds
1 tablespoon maca powder
2 tablespoons coconut oil
1 teaspoon sea salt

Place the almonds in a food processor, nut grinder, or high-speed blender and grind into a flour, about 30 seconds. Add the rest of the ingredients and blend for about 10 minutes, stopping the machine to scrape down the sides as needed. Blend until your perfect crunchy-to-creamy ratio is achieved.

Store in an airtight glass container in the refrigerator for up to 2 weeks.

KITCHEN NOTE

To help the nut butter come together in the blender, add 1 tablespoon of melted coconut oil at a time until smooth.

✦ ✦ ✦ ✦

JUICY JAMS 3 WAYS

With just a little maple syrup and chia seeds at their core, the following nutritionally dense jams use the abundance of colors, flavors, and natural sugars in berries, tropical fruits, and dried fruits to make deliciously flavorful sweet spreads that are low on the glycemic index. Without the processed, refined sugar that steals the nutrients and hydration from your skin, you may begin to see a clearer complexion and a healthier weight.

TROPICAL MARMALADE
MAKES 2½ CUPS

1 cup pineapple (see directions)
1 cup mango (see directions)
1 cup passion fruit (see directions)
2 tablespoons chia seeds
1 to 2 tablespoons pure maple syrup

Remove the stems, pits, seeds, and skin from the fruits and chop the flesh into small pieces. Combine all the ingredients in a blender and process until smooth. Alternatively, if you prefer a chunkier jam, mash the flesh with a fork until pulpy and juicy, then mix in the rest of the ingredients.

Add additional chia seeds, 1 teaspoon at a time, for a thicker jam.

3 cups mixed berries
2 tablespoons chia seeds
2 tablespoons fresh lemon juice
1 to 2 tablespoons pure maple syrup

Combine all the ingredients in a blender and blend until smooth. Alternatively, if you prefer a chunkier jam, mash the berries with a fork until pulpy and juicy, then mix in the rest of the ingredients.

Add additional chia seeds, 1 teaspoon at a time, for a thicker jam.

Cooked method:

If you prefer to cook your jams on the stovetop, transfer the fruit mixture to a saucepan and set over medium heat. Mash the fruit with the back of a fork. Simmer for 5 to 10 minutes, until the fruit begins to break down.

Remove from the heat and stir in the maple syrup, lemon juice, and chia seeds. Allow to cool and set for 15 minutes. If you prefer a thicker consistency, stir in more chia seeds, 1 teaspoon at a time. If you prefer a smoother jam, simply process in a blender for a few seconds until smooth.

Store in an airtight glass container in the refrigerator for up to 2 weeks.

APRICOT AND FIG SPREAD
MAKES 2½ CUPS

¾ cup dried figs
¾ cup dried apricots
1 cup fresh orange juice
2 teaspoons orange zest
½ teaspoon pure vanilla extract

Chop the figs and apricots into small chunks, place in a bowl, top with the orange juice, and soak for 1 hour. Combine all the ingredients, including the orange juice, in a blender and process until smooth.

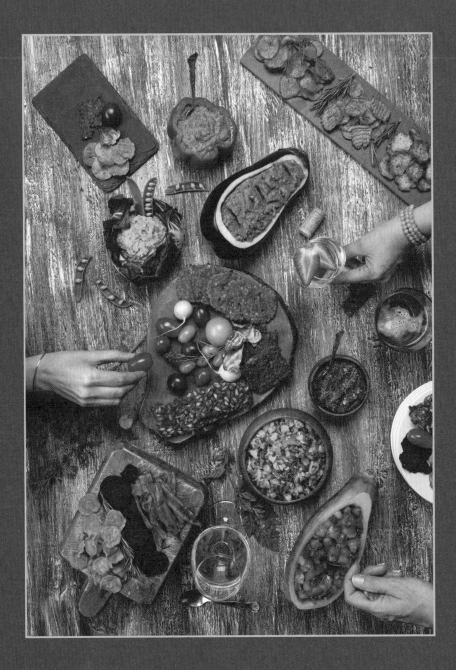

SUPERCHARGED SNACKS

Chips, Crisps, Dips, and Salsas

We are all designed to eat in a grazing fashion. No wonder we love our snacks! Stock your kitchen with these healthful versions of your favorite goodies and elevate your snacking game.

Vegetable Chips

Smoked Carrot Bacon

Mediterranean Crisps

Peppery Apricot Thins

3-Seed Crackers

Nettle and Hemp Seed Pesto

Chunky Guacamole with Tomatillos

Strawberry Papaya Goji Salsa

Smoky Eggplant Caviar

Muhammara Red Pepper Walnut Dip

Green Pea and Mint Hummus with Spirulina Oil Drizzle

VEGETABLE CHIPS

Loaded with beautifying, mineral-rich vegetables, this all-purpose chip recipe is all about options: use the listed ingredients or choose your favorite veggies to play with.

MAKES 3 TO 4 CUPS

1 sweet potato, peeled
1 blue potato, peeled
1 parsnip, peeled
1 jicama, peeled
1 red beet, peeled
1 golden beet, peeled
1 tablespoon olive oil
1 teaspoon fresh rosemary
1 teaspoon red pepper flakes
Sea salt
Freshly ground black pepper

Preheat the oven to 325°F.

Slice the vegetables into thin disks, using a mandoline, or finely slice by hand.

Pat the vegetables dry and place them in a bowl along with the olive oil, rosemary, red pepper flakes, and salt and black pepper to taste. Turn to coat evenly and transfer to a baking sheet in a single layer.

Bake for 20 minutes, or until golden and crispy, keeping a close eye on your chips after the 15-minute point as some may cook faster than others. Remove from the oven and let cool.

KITCHEN NOTE

If you prefer to make the vegetable chips in a dehydrator, spread the raw, uncoated vegetables in a single layer on the trays of the device and dehydrate for 10 hours at the 125 level setting or until crispy. Just before serving, toss the chips in the seasoned oil.

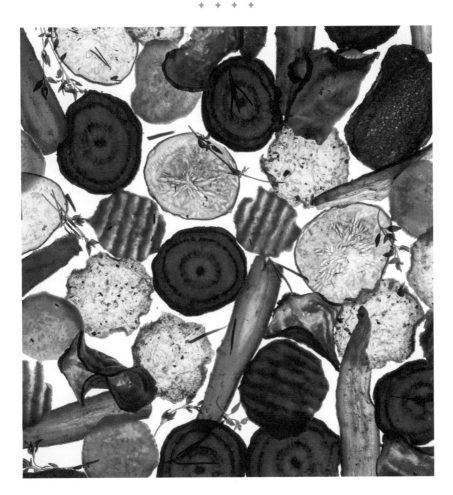

SMOKED CARROT BACON

With a balance of crunchy and chewy—and loads of baconlike smokiness—these smoked carrot strips are the perfect addition to your sandwiches or you can chop them into bite-size bits and sprinkle on scrambles, chowders, and chili.

MAKES 1 TO 2 CUPS

4 medium carrots, peeled
2 tablespoons cold-pressed olive oil
1 tablespoon tamari (or coconut aminos, for a soy-free option)
½ teaspoon chipotle chile powder
1 teaspoon liquid smoke (optional)

Preheat the oven to 325°F.

Slice the carrots into long strips, using a mandoline or peeler, or thinly slice by hand.

Mix all the remaining ingredients together in a small bowl. Using a pastry brush, coat the sliced carrots on both sides. Transfer the carrot slices to a baking sheet in a single layer.

Bake for 20 minutes, or until golden and crispy. Remove from the oven and let cool.

✦ ✦ ✦ ✦

BEAUTY FOOD SPOTLIGHT

Carrots contain high doses of vitamin A, vitamin C, and numerous antioxidants that aid in the production of collagen, a protein vital in maintaining skin elasticity. Plus, carotenoids in carrots protects the skin against the sun's harsh rays by acting as a natural sunblock.

✦ ✦ ✦ ✦

MEDITERRANEAN CRISPS

These delicious savory crisps are entirely grain free. Made with nuts and seeds, these skin-loving crisps are rich in vitamin E, our body's main fat-soluble antioxidant. This incredibly anti-inflammatory vitamin helps reduce the risk of inflammatory skin conditions, including acne, eczema, and psoriasis.

MAKES 40

2 cups cashews

⅔ cup flaxseeds

⅔ cup almond flour

½ teaspoon baking soda

2 tablespoons olive oil

2 tablespoons miso paste

1½ cups sun-dried tomatoes, soaked in water, drained, and then minced

½ cup minced fresh herbs

¼ cup water

Preheat the oven to 350°F. Line two baking sheets with parchment paper.

Place the cashews and flaxseeds in a food processor and grind into a fine powder. Add the almond flour and baking soda and pulse to combine. Add the olive oil, miso, sun-dried tomatoes, herbs, and water (see Kitchen Note) and process until a uniform dough is formed. Remove the dough from the food processor and allow to sit for 15 minutes.

Divide the dough in half. Place one portion of the dough onto one of the prepared baking sheets. Cover with an additional piece of parchment paper and, using a rolling pin, roll out the dough to cover the entire surface. With a knife, cut the dough into twenty squares. Repeat on the other prepared baking sheet with the other portion of dough.

(continued)

Bake both sheets for 15 minutes before flipping the crackers over. Continue to bake for another 10 minutes, or until golden.

Remove from the oven and let the crackers cool on the pan. Store in a sealed container for up to 2 weeks.

+ + + +

KITCHEN NOTE

When blending your dough, check its consistency. It should be sticky and pliable. Start with less water, and if the dough is too dry, mix in additional water, 1 teaspoon at a time.

+ + + +

PEPPERY APRICOT THINS

These seedy crisps, with their beautifying dose of protein, fiber, and healthy fat, are full of B vitamins and iron that support energy levels, and essential fatty acids that encourage smooth, soft skin. These sweet and peppery chewy thins are satisfyingly delicious.

MAKES ABOUT 20

1 cup chopped dried apricots
1 cup water
2 cups raw pistachios
½ cup flaxseed meal
2 tablespoons peppercorns, crushed
½ teaspoon sea salt

Preheat the oven to 350°F. Line a baking sheet with parchment paper.

Combine the dried apricots and water in a blender and blend into a paste.

Place the pistachios in a food processor and pulse until finely chopped.

Add the remaining ingredients, including the apricot paste, to the pistachios and pulse until combined.

Roll out the mixture to ¼-inch thickness on the prepared baking sheet, and with a knife, cut the dough into twenty squares. Alternatively, you can use a cookie cutter to form rounds. Bake in the center rack of the oven for 20 minutes, or until the crackers are golden. Remove from the oven and let cool on the baking sheet.

Stored in a sealed container, the crackers will last for several weeks.

(continued)

KITCHEN NOTE

If using a dehydrator, dehydrate the mixture at 115°F for 4 hours, flip the sheets, peel off the dehydrator sheet, place the mixture dried side up on the dehydrator screens, and continue to dehydrate for 4 more hours, or until dry.

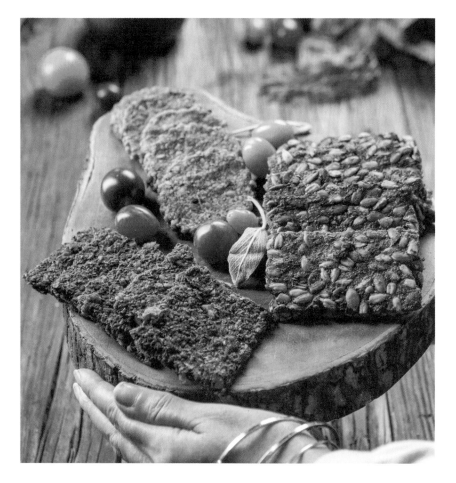

3-SEED CRACKERS

These protein-rich savory crisps packed with sunflower seeds, pumpkin seeds, and flaxseeds, are high in tryptophan, an amino acid that can reduce stress and cravings for sugary treats, which can age your skin. The fiber will help you feel full longer.

MAKES 40

1 cup sunflower seeds
½ cup pumpkin seeds
1 cup flaxseeds
½ cup almond flour
½ teaspoon baking soda
½ cup minced white onion
3 tablespoons minced garlic
2 tablespoons olive oil
2 tablespoons miso paste
¼ cup filtered water
2 tablespoons various seeds, for garnish

Preheat the oven to 350°F. Line two baking sheets with parchment paper.

Place the sunflower seeds, pumpkin seeds, and flaxseeds in a food processor and grind into a fine powder. Add the almond flour and baking soda and pulse to combine. Add the onion, garlic, oil, miso, and water and process until a uniform dough is formed. Add the seed mixture reserved for garnish and mix briefly to combine, leaving a textured surface. Remove the dough from the food processor and allow to sit for 15 minutes.

Divide the dough in half. Place one portion of the dough on one of the prepared baking sheets. Cover with an additional piece of parchment paper and,

(continued)

using a rolling pin, roll out the dough to cover the entire surface. With a knife, cut the dough into twenty squares. Repeat on the second prepared baking sheet with the other portion of dough.

Bake both sheets for 15 minutes before flipping the crackers over. Continue to bake for another 10 minutes, or until golden.

Remove from the oven and let the crackers cool on the pan. Store in a sealed container for up to 2 weeks.

NETTLE AND HEMP SEED PESTO

Earthy and bright, this nettle pesto is made with omega-rich hemp seeds. Nettle resembles spinach in flavor and is an incredible source of vitamins A and C, protein, and iron. With its nourishing, diuretic, and anti-inflammatory properties, nettle is a natural hair and skin beautifier that has been shown to clear up acne and encourage thicker, shinier hair growth.

MAKES 1¼ CUPS

3 garlic cloves, peeled
2 cups packed nettle leaves
1 cup fresh basil leaves
¾ cup hemp seeds
2 tablespoons fresh lemon juice
¼ cup flaxseed oil
Sea salt and freshly ground black pepper
⅓ cup nutritional yeast (optional)

Place the garlic in a food processor and process until minced. Turn off the processor. Add the nettle leaves, basil, hemp seeds, lemon juice, and salt and pepper to taste. Turn on the processor again and drizzle in the oil. Process until the pesto reaches your desired consistency, stopping to scrape down the sides as necessary. Taste and add more lemon juice, salt, or pepper as desired.

Transfer the mixture to a serving bowl and serve at room temperature. Store the pesto in an airtight glass container in the refrigerator for up to 1 week.

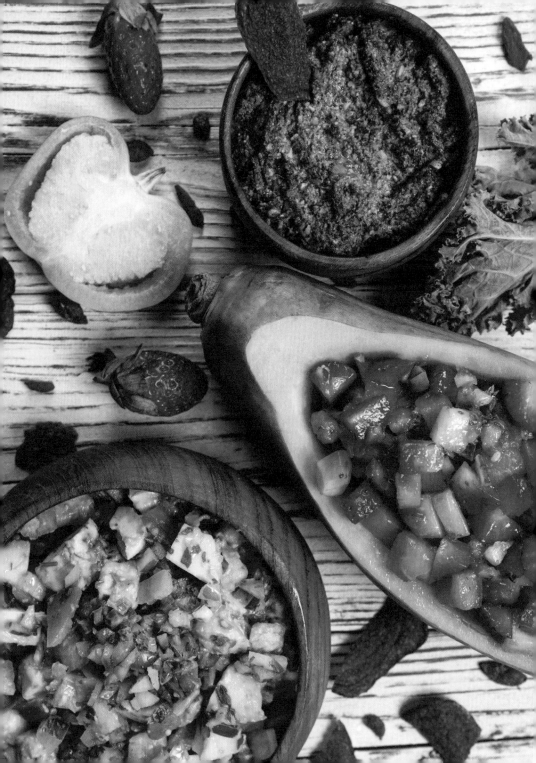

CHUNKY GUACAMOLE
WITH TOMATILLOS

In addition to avocado's skin-loving fats, this guacamole sneaks in mineral-
and protein-rich wheatgrass.

MAKES 4 CUPS

3 cups peeled, pitted, and diced avocado
1 cup diced tomatillo
¼ cup fresh lemon juice
½ cup chopped fresh cilantro, plus more for garnish
¼ cup minced red onion
2 garlic cloves, minced
½ fresh red chile, seeded and minced
2 tablespoons olive oil
Sea salt and freshly ground black pepper
1 teaspoon wheatgrass powder (optional)

Place the avocado in a medium bowl and roughly mash the avocados, using the
back of a fork, leaving some texture. Add the remaining ingredients and stir to
combine. Adjust the seasoning to taste. Transfer to a serving bowl and garnish
with extra cilantro. Serve immediately.

✦ ✦ ✦ ✦

BEAUTY FOOD SPOTLIGHT

*Highly alkalizing, wheatgrass can stabilize an unbalanced pH, detoxify
the body, and normalize the thyroid for a balanced metabolism. Made of
70 percent chlorophyll, wheatgrass is also an important blood builder.*

✦ ✦ ✦ ✦

STRAWBERRY PAPAYA GOJI SALSA

Sweet, savory, and fresh, this superfood salsa encourages collagen production, protects skin from oxidative stress, and maintains skin's elasticity.

MAKES 3½ CUPS

¼ cup goji berries
3 tablespoons fresh lime juice
2 cups peeled, seeded, and chopped ripe papaya
1 cup hulled and chopped strawberries
¼ cup finely chopped red onion
1 green jalapeño pepper, seeded and finely chopped
2 tablespoons olive oil
Sea salt and freshly ground black pepper

Soak the goji berries in the lime juice in a medium bowl for 15 minutes.

Toss all the ingredients together, including the gojis and the lime juice. Transfer to a serving bowl, cover, and chill for 30 minutes before serving.

✦ ✦ ✦ ✦

BEAUTY FOOD SPOTLIGHT

Rich in vitamin C, beta-carotene, and amino acids, goji berries help you maintain a smooth, radiant complexion by increasing blood circulation, soothing redness, and reducing inflammation.

✦ ✦ ✦ ✦

SMOKY EGGPLANT CAVIAR

Thick and delicious, eggplant caviar, or baba ghanoush, is a delicious dip or spread that calls for eggplant at its base. This version omits the mayo and includes lots of additional fresh herbs, spices, and chia seeds for an extra-nutritious punch.

MAKES 2½ CUPS

2 medium (1 pound each) eggplants
2 medium tomatoes, chopped
2 tablespoons olive oil
2 tablespoons fresh lemon juice
3 garlic cloves
1 white onion
1 chipotle pepper
1 tablespoon chopped fresh parsley
1 tablespoon chopped fresh mint
1 tablespoon chia seeds (optional)
Sea salt and freshly ground black pepper

Preheat the oven to 400°F. Place the eggplants on a baking sheet and prick the surface of each eggplant with a knife several times. Bake for 30 minutes, or until tender. Remove from the oven and let cool.

Peel away the skins and scoop the flesh into the bowl of a food processor.

Add the rest of the ingredients, including salt and black pepper to taste, and process until the mixture reaches your desired consistency. Taste and add more lemon juice, oil, salt, or black pepper as desired.

(continued)

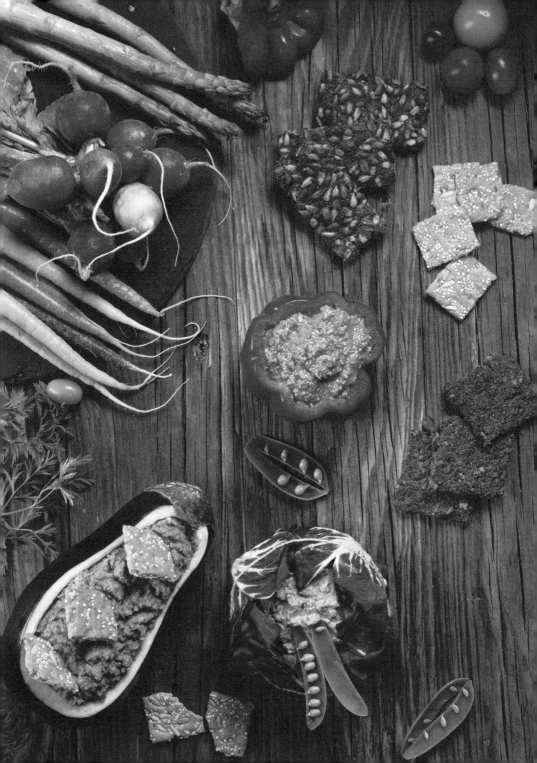

To serve, transfer the mixture to a bowl, sprinkle with chopped fresh herbs, and serve with warm pita wedges or crisps.

Store the caviar in an airtight glass container in the refrigerator for up to 1 week.

✦ ✦ ✦ ✦

BEAUTY FOOD SPOTLIGHT

Rich in antioxidants and antibacterial and antiviral properties, eggplants are an important supporter of timeless, toned skin. The anthocyanin pigments, in particular, nourish healthy collagen for improved skin elasticity and antiaging benefits.

✦ ✦ ✦ ✦

MUHAMMARA RED PEPPER WALNUT DIP

Loaded with nutrients, proteins, and healthy fats, this delicious Middle Eastern spread is full of skin-nourishing benefits.

MAKES 2½ CUPS

½ cup olive oil

4 large fresh red bell peppers, ribs and seeds removed, diced

1 onion, diced

3 garlic cloves, minced

2 tablespoons fresh lemon juice

1 teaspoon ground cumin

½ teaspoon red pepper flakes

2 cup walnuts, chopped, plus more for garnish

Sea salt and freshly ground black pepper

Heat the oil in a large saucepan over medium-low heat. Cook the onion and garlic, stirring frequently, for 4 minutes, or until they begin to soften. Add the bell peppers, cover, and cook, stirring occasionally for 10 to 15 minutes, until softened.

Place the remaining ingredients, except the olive oil, in a food processor or blender and process until the mixture is smooth. With the motor still running, gradually pour in the olive oil. Add the cooked ingredients and process until the mixture reaches your desired consistency. Taste and adjust the lemon juice, oil, salt and black pepper as desired.

To serve, transfer the mixture to a bowl and garnish with crushed walnuts. Store the muhammara in an airtight glass container in the refrigerator for up to 1 week.

+ + + +

BEAUTY FOOD SPOTLIGHT

Red bell peppers are a great source of vitamin C, which keeps our locks strong and healthy. Vitamin C helps the body use non-heme iron, the type found in plant foods, ensuring that there is enough iron in our red blood cells to carry oxygen to hair follicles. Even minor vitamin C deficiencies can lead to dry, splitting hair that breaks easily.

+ + + +

GREEN PEA AND MINT HUMMUS WITH SPIRULINA OIL DRIZZLE

This fresh, playful green hummus is nutrient dense and high in protein. Top with a drizzle of the phytonutrient-rich spirulina oil for healthful bonus points.

MAKES 1½ CUPS

Hummus

2 cups fresh green peas, cooked and cooled
2 tablespoons fresh lemon juice
¼ cup hemp oil or olive oil
2 tablespoons tahini
2 garlic cloves, peeled and chopped
2 tablespoons chopped fresh mint
Sea salt and freshly ground black pepper

Spirulina oil

1 tablespoon olive oil
¼ teaspoon spirulina powder

To make the hummus:
Combine all the hummus ingredients a high-speed blender and blend until smooth. Adjust the seasonings to taste.

To make the spirulina oil:

Whisk together the olive oil and spirulina powder in a small bowl.

Transfer the hummus to a serving dish and drizzle with the spirulina oil.

Store in an airtight glass container in the refrigerator for up to 3 days.

✦ ✦ ✦ ✦

BEAUTY FOOD SPOTLIGHT

*Peas contain great amounts of fiber that support natural detox,
keep us fuller longer, help us release a steady flow of energy,
and improve weight loss.*

✦ ✦ ✦ ✦

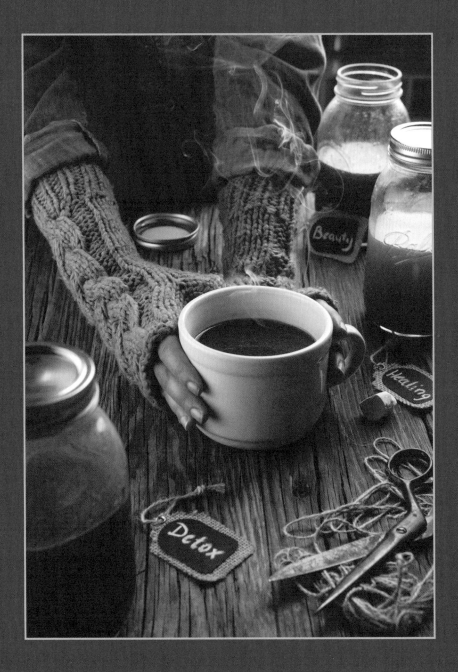

A CUP OF COMFORT

Medicinal Broths, Soups, and Stews

There's something truly comforting about soups. A simmering pot feeds both your appetite and your soul, detoxifying, alkalizing, and restoring body and spirit. On the following pages you'll first find three medicinal broths followed by traditional soups with mineral-rich nutrients that will nurture and beautify. The medicinal broths can be sipped on their own or used as the base to many of the soup recipes that follow.

Vegetable Beauty Broth

Seaweed Detox Broth

Healing Mushroom Broth

Creamy Pumpkin and Roasted Chestnut Bisque

Thai Noodle Nourish Bowl

Mushroom Chowder

Healing Kale and Lentil Dal Stew

Roasted Red Pepper and Hibiscus Soup

Green Gazpacho

Chilled Honeydew and Fennel Soup

VEGETABLE BEAUTY BROTH

Enjoy nature's best beauty nutrients in this powerful broth. Thanks to an abundance of anti-inflammatory nutrients and antioxidants in the vegetables and goji berries, this warm beauty drink fights free radicals and supplies electrolytes for cellular hydration, while functional ingredients, including garlic, chile, ginger, and turmeric, help boost circulation that aids in nutrient absorption. Feel free to customize your broth by using your preferred vegetables.

MAKES 6 CUPS

3 tablespoons extra-virgin olive oil
1 cup chopped onion
1 cup chopped carrot
1 cup chopped parsnip
1 cup chopped celery
4 garlic cloves, chopped
1 small chile pepper
1 (1-inch) piece fresh ginger, chopped
1 (1-inch) piece fresh turmeric, chopped
1 tablespoon raw apple cider vinegar
8 cups filtered water
1½ teaspoons peppercorns
3 bay leaves
3 sprigs fresh thyme
3 sprigs fresh parsley
¼ cup goji berries
Sea salt and freshly ground black pepper

Heat the oil in a large pot over medium heat. Add the onion, carrot, parsnip, celery, garlic, chile pepper, ginger, and turmeric and cook for 5 minutes, stirring frequently. Stir in the vinegar and add the water. Bring to a boil and add the peppercorns, bay leaves, thyme, parsley, and goji berries. Lower the heat and simmer, partly covered, for 1 hour. Strain the broth and discard the vegetables. Add salt and black pepper to taste.

Let the broth cool and store in an airtight glass container in the refrigerator for up to 1 week. Use the broth in the soup recipes or enjoy on its own.

✦　✦　✦　✦

KITCHEN NOTE

For a balanced flavor, I use a standard mirepoix of onion, carrot, parsnip, and celery. But beyond that, I encourage you to get creative.

✦　✦　✦　✦

SEAWEED DETOX BROTH

Forget the cleanse and reach for a cup of this incredibly powerful mineralizing broth. Rich in protein and amino acids to help the body fight infections, and fiber that encourages the growth of good bacteria in the gut, seaweed also helps detox our body by protecting the liver from toxic damage and encouraging healthy cellular function.

There are literally thousands of sea vegetable varieties. I encourage you to choose your favorites and discover new ones, to maximize the nutrients and customize your broth.

MAKES 6 CUPS

3 tablespoons extra-virgin olive oil
½ cup chopped onion
½ cup chopped carrots
½ cup chopped parsnip
½ cup chopped celery
2 garlic cloves, chopped
1 teaspoon red pepper flakes
8 cups filtered water
1 cup sea vegetables: dulse, wakame, kelp, or kombu
3 tablespoons chickpea miso paste
Sea salt and freshly ground black pepper

Heat the oil in a large pot over medium heat. Add the onion, carrot, parsnip, celery, garlic, and red pepper flakes and cook for 5 minutes, stirring frequently. Add the water and bring to a boil. Stir in the sea vegetables and lower the heat to medium-low. Simmer, partly covered, for 1 hour.

Remove from the heat, strain the broth, and discard the vegetables. Stir in the miso paste and salt and pepper to taste.

Let cool and store in an airtight glass container in the refrigerator for up to 1 week. Use the broth in the soup recipes or enjoy on its own.

✦ ✦ ✦ ✦

KITCHEN NOTE

Use the drained, cooked seaweed as a delicious addition to soups, salads, and bowls.

✦ ✦ ✦ ✦

HEALING MUSHROOM BROTH

This warm restorative mushroom tonic works with your body on every level. The beta-glucan fibers found in the cell walls of mushrooms are known to stimulate the immune system and to help prevent disease. In fact, many mushrooms have long been used throughout Asia for medicinal purposes. This rich, earthy healing broth supplies phytochemicals for adrenal support and helps with cellular recovery and stress management.

Since there are more than 270 species of mushroom known to have unique therapeutic properties, feel free to use a variety of dried and fresh mushrooms and any medicinal powdered favorites you might have, to customize your broth.

MAKES 6 CUPS

2 ounces dried shiitake or maitake mushrooms (these contain powerful immune-boosting properties)

8 cups filtered water

3 tablespoons extra-virgin olive oil

1 cup chopped onion

1 cup chopped carrot

1 cup chopped parsnip

1 cup chopped celery

4 garlic cloves, chopped

2 sprigs fresh rosemary

3 sprigs fresh parsley

1½ teaspoons peppercorns

3 bay leaves

1 tablespoon raw apple cider vinegar

1 cup fresh mushrooms

Sea salt and freshly ground black pepper

Soak the dried mushrooms in 1 cup of the filtered water in a glass bowl for 30 minutes.

Heat the oil in a large pot over medium heat. Add the onion, carrot, parsnip, celery, garlic, and fresh mushrooms and cook for 5 minutes, stirring frequently. Mix in the dried mushrooms along with their soaking liquid and add the vinegar and remaining 7 cups of filtered water. Bring to a boil. Add the peppercorns, bay leaves, rosemary, and parsley. Lower the heat and simmer, partly covered, for 1 hour.

Remove from the heat, strain the broth, and discard the vegetables. Add salt and pepper to taste.

Let cool and store in an airtight glass container in the refrigerator for up to 1 week. Use the broth in the soup recipes or enjoy on its own.

✦ ✦ ✦ ✦

KITCHEN TIP

Use the strained, cooked veggies to make a delicious pâté. Simply blend them with ½ cup of walnuts plus some favorite herbs and spices.

✦ ✦ ✦ ✦

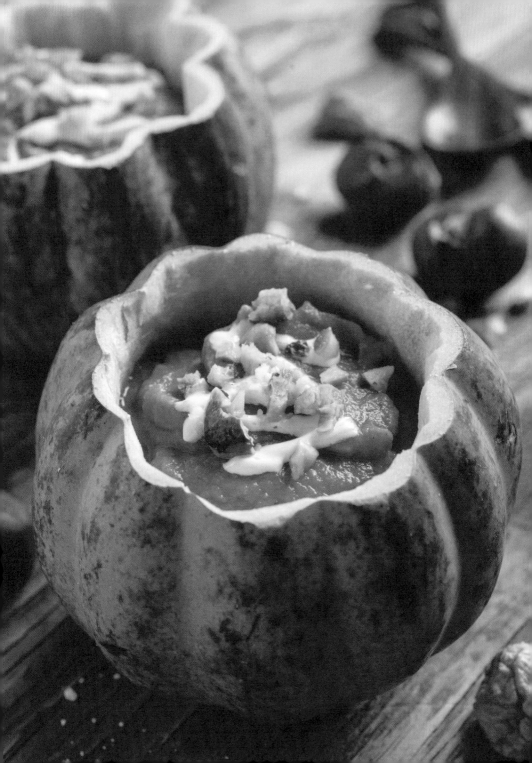

CREAMY PUMPKIN AND ROASTED CHESTNUT BISQUE

Healthy, satisfying, and perfect for chillier weather, this wonderfully complex soup will nurture you inside and out. The high concentration of vitamin C and antioxidant compounds in chestnuts make them an ideal addition to this immunity-boosting recipe.

SERVES: 4 TO 6

1 medium (2–3 pounds) pumpkin or 2 cups pure pumpkin puree

2 tablespoons coconut oil, plus more for brushing pumpkin, if using

1 small red onion, chopped

1 carrot, peeled and chopped

2 garlic cloves, minced

2 cups Vegetable Beauty Broth (page 78)

1½ cups peeled roasted chestnuts

2 cups canned coconut milk

¼ teaspoon sea salt

¼ teaspoon freshly ground black pepper

¼ teaspoon ground cinnamon

¼ teaspoon grated nutmeg

Sweet Cream, for serving (page 203)

If using fresh pumpkin, preheat the oven to 375°F and line a baking sheet with parchment paper. Cut the pumpkin in half and remove the seeds and strings. Brush the flesh with oil, season with sea salt and black pepper, and place face down on the baking sheet. Roast in the oven for 45 to 50 minutes, until the

(continued)

skin begins to brown and the flesh is tender. Remove from the oven and let cool for 10 minutes, then peel away the skin and set the pumpkin aside.

Heat the oil in a large saucepan over medium heat. Add the onion, carrot, and garlic and cook for 5 minutes, stirring frequently. Add the broth, pumpkin, and chestnuts and bring to a boil. Lower the heat to medium-low, add the coconut milk, salt, and spices, and simmer for 20 minutes.

Transfer the soup mixture to a blender and puree until smooth.

Taste and adjust the seasonings as needed. To serve, pour the soup into serving bowls and swirl the sweet cream on top.

Store in an airtight glass container in the refrigerator for up to 3 days.

✦ ✦ ✦ ✦

KITCHEN NOTES

Roasting your own chestnuts is a wonderful winter tradition that makes the whole house smell like the holidays. Here's how:
Preheat the oven to 400°F. Score an X into the shell of each chestnut and evenly spread them on a dry baking sheet. Drizzle with olive oil and roast until tender, about 45 minutes. Remove from the oven and allow to cool. Peel and enjoy.
Although fresh is always best, to save time, you can use two 15-ounce cans of organic pumpkin instead of roasting.

✦ ✦ ✦ ✦

THAI NOODLE NOURISH BOWL

This mineral-rich soup is the perfect balance of savory, salty, and spicy, plus it's fully customizable. You can vary the toppings as well as the noodles to give this soup your own personal flair.

SERVES 4 TO 6

Soup
4 cups Seaweed Detox Broth (page 80)
2 lemongrass stalks, sliced
1 (4-inch) piece fresh ginger, sliced
2 teaspoons chile paste
¼ cup fresh lime juice
Sea salt and freshly ground black pepper

Kelp noodles
1 (12-ounce) package kelp noodles
1½ cups warm water
1 teaspoon baking soda

Optional garnishes
Edamame
Mushrooms
Bok choy
Mung bean sprouts
Fresh mint
Fresh cilantro
Fresh Thai basil
Green onion, sliced thinly
Sweet red pepper, sliced thinly

(continued)

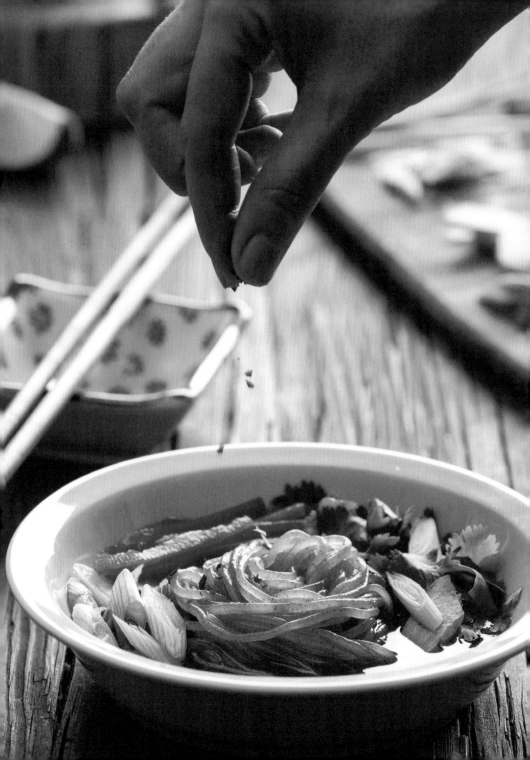

To make the soup:

Combine the seaweed broth, ginger, lemongrass, and chile paste in a large pot over high heat. Bring the mixture to a boil. Lower the heat to a low simmer and cook for 15 minutes.

To make the noodles:

While the broth is simmering, prepare the kelp noodles. Thoroughly rinse them, then soak the noodles in water and baking soda for 15 minutes. Rinse well.

Add the noodles and the lime juice to the simmering soup. Remove from the heat and let the soup sit for 5 minutes.

To serve, divide the noodles in serving bowls and pour the soup on top. Arrange your desired garnish in sections or stir together.

Store in an airtight glass container in the refrigerator for up to 2 days.

+ + + +

KITCHEN NOTE

This is an extremely versatile recipe. You can replace the kelp noodles with buckwheat or rice noodles or even quinoa, buckwheat, or black rice, for an interesting twist.

BEAUTY FOOD SPOTLIGHT

Made from a brown seaweed that grows in deep waters, kelp noodles are a nutritional powerhouse, full of calcium, iron, and vitamin K. They are also an incredible source of iodine, essential for proper thyroid function, a healthy metabolism, and weight loss.

+ + + +

MUSHROOM CHOWDER

With chunks of melt-away potatoes, savory mushrooms, and aromatic rosemary, this creamy, wholesome chowder supports the immune system and increases skin hydration and skin elasticity.

SERVES 4 TO 6

2 tablespoons extra-virgin olive oil
1 cup thinly sliced leek, well rinsed
½ cup chopped celery
4 garlic cloves, minced
3 cups chopped mixed mushrooms
2 cups diced red potato
1 sprig fresh rosemary
4 cups almond milk
2 cups Healing Mushroom broth (page 82)
Sea salt and freshly ground black pepper
Chopped fresh herbs or bits of Smoked Carrot Bacon (page 58), for garnish

Heat the oil in a large pot over medium heat. Add the leek, celery, garlic, and mushrooms and cook for 10 minutes. Add the potato, rosemary, and mushroom broth. Bring the mixture to a boil over high heat, then cover the pot and lower the heat to medium-low. Simmer for 30 minutes, until the potato is tender. Discard the rosemary sprig.

Add the almond milk and simmer for an additional 5 minutes. Season to taste with salt and pepper.

To serve, ladle the chowder into bowls and sprinkle with fresh chopped herbs or smoked carrot bacon bits.

Store in an airtight glass container in the refrigerator for up to 2 days.

KITCHEN NOTE

Because of their porous nature, mushrooms have the tendency to easily absorb chemicals from the soil in which they're grown. As much as possible, choose to purchase organic.

✦ ✦ ✦ ✦

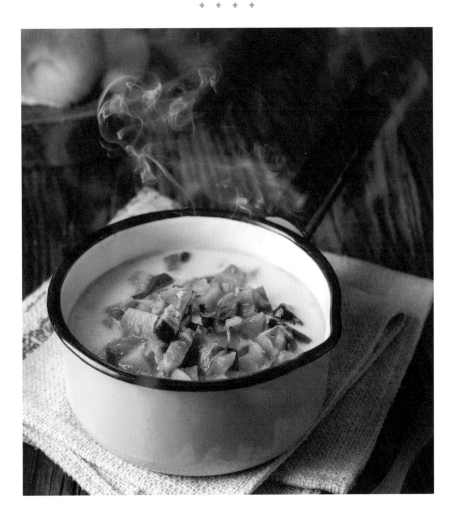

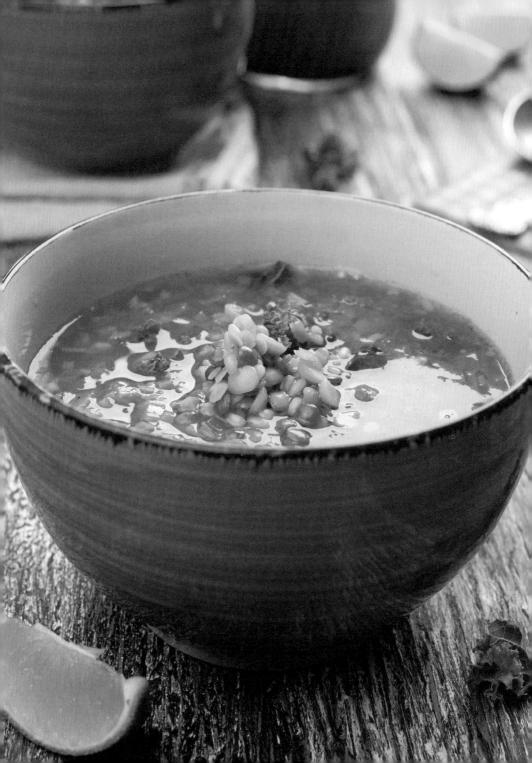

HEALING KALE AND LENTIL DAL STEW

The lentils in this feel-good stew simply melt away into a creamy, comforting bowl of goodness. Hearty and comforting, this fiber-rich dish helps lower cholesterol and regulate blood sugar essential for healthy skin aging.

SERVES 4 TO 6

2 cups dried lentils
1 tablespoon coconut oil
1 cup finely diced yellow onion
4 garlic cloves, minced
1 (1-inch) piece fresh ginger, peeled and grated
1 teaspoon ground turmeric
1 teaspoon ground cumin
1 teaspoon ground coriander
½ teaspoon red pepper flakes
½ teaspoon garam masala (optional)
4 cups Vegetable Beauty Broth (page 78)
1 cup chopped kale
3 tablespoons fresh lemon juice
Sea salt and freshly ground black pepper
Chopped fresh parsley, for garnish

Rinse the lentils with cold water and let drain.

Heat the oil in a large pot over medium heat. Add the onion, garlic, and ginger and cook for 5 minutes, stirring frequently.

(continued)

Add the lentils, turmeric, cumin, coriander, red pepper flakes, and garam masala, if using. Stir to combine. Pour in the broth and bring to boil. Lower the heat to medium-low and let simmer for 30 minutes, or until the lentils are tender.

Remove from the heat and stir in the kale and lemon juice. Season to taste with salt and black pepper.

To serve, ladle the stew into bowls, and top with chopped fresh parsley. Store in an airtight glass container in the refrigerator for up to 2 days.

✦ ✦ ✦ ✦

KITCHEN NOTE

To ensure that its nutrition isn't destroyed through heat, add the kale at the very end of the cooking.

✦ ✦ ✦ ✦

ROASTED RED PEPPER AND HIBISCUS SOUP

The stunning hibiscus flower lends its color and flavor to the base of this crimson creation also colored by red bell peppers. Loaded with antioxidants and folic acid, this soup is truly fabulous for promoting glowing skin. For a fun variation, try this soup chilled on hot summer days.

SERVES 4 TO 6

8 large red bell peppers
4 hibiscus tea bags
4 cups boiling water
2 tablespoons olive oil
1 cup chopped red onion
2 garlic cloves, chopped
2 teaspoons lime juice
1 tablespoon chopped basil
Sea salt and freshly ground black pepper
Sour Cream (page 202), for garnish

Preheat the oven to 400°F. Place the bell peppers on a foil-lined baking sheet and roast in the oven for 30 minutes, until the skins blister and char. Remove from the oven and transfer the peppers to a glass bowl. Cover with plastic wrap and let sit for 30 minutes.

When the peppers are completely cool, pull out the cores and seeds and peel away the charred skins over a large bowl to catch the juice. Set the pepper flesh and juices aside.

(continued)

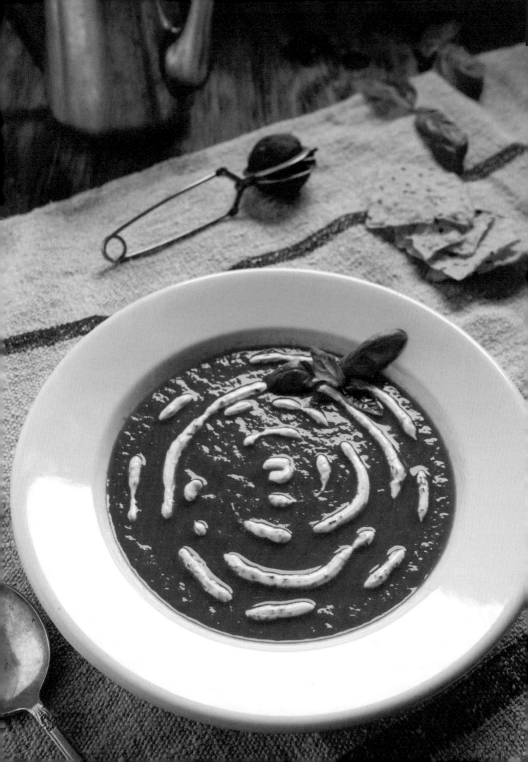

Steep the hibiscus tea in the boiling water for 15 minutes and discard the tea bags.

Heat the oil in a large saucepan over medium heat. Add the onion and garlic and cook for 5 minutes, stirring frequently. Add the tea infusion and red peppers and bring to a boil. Lower the heat to medium-low and simmer for 20 minutes.

Transfer the soup mixture to a blender, add the lime juice and basil, and puree the soup until smooth. Taste, and adjust the seasonings as needed. To serve, pour the soup into serving bowls and swirl the sour cream on top.

Store in an airtight glass container in the refrigerator for up to 3 days.

+ + + +

KITCHEN NOTES

This recipe is a great example of the power of using tea to create unexpected flavorful broths in the healthiest of ways. In Japan, ochazuke, green tea over rice, has been enjoyed for centuries. Although fresh is always best, to save time, you can use 4 cups of jarred organic roasted peppers instead of roasting.

+ + + +

GREEN GAZPACHO

This green beauty practically glows with copious amounts of vitamins C and E, zinc, and silica, a beauty trace mineral responsible for strong connective tissue and healthy skin.

Serve this bright and creamy soup straight from the blender during the warm summer months, for a refreshing yet nourishing meal.

SERVES 4 TO 6

1 cup seeded and chopped green bell pepper
1 cup chopped tomatillos
2 garlic cloves
1 cup chopped cucumber
½ green chile, seeded
½ cup fresh cilantro
¼ cup fresh mint
1 cup pitted and peeled avocado
¼ cup chives, topped and tailed
½ cup lime juice
Sea salt and freshly ground black pepper
Avocado oil, for garnish

Place all the ingredients, except the salt, black pepper, and avocado oil, in a blender and blend. Taste, and season as desired. If you prefer a lighter soup, add water to achieve your desired consistency. Chill for 30 minutes before serving. Pour into bowls and top with a drizzle of avocado oil.

Store in an airtight glass container in the refrigerator for up to 2 days.

KITCHEN NOTE

*Because flavors become muted in cold dishes, season this gazpacho as
you go and taste again after chilling.*

CHILLED HONEYDEW AND FENNEL SOUP

Sweet, bright, and refreshing with just a hint of spice, this lovely chilled soup comes together in a flash, perfect for long, lazy summer days. And your skin will thank you for its natural beauty-promoting vitamins and minerals.

SERVES 4 TO 6

4 cups seeded and roughly chopped honeydew melon
1 cup roughly chopped fennel
4 cups roughly chopped cucumber
¼ cup aloe water
½ cup fresh lemon juice
½ green chile pepper, finely chopped
Sea salt and freshly ground black pepper
Fennel fronds, for garnish
3 tablespoons extra-virgin olive oil or avocado oil, for garnish

Place the melon, fennel, cucumber, aloe water, lemon juice, chile pepper, and salt in a high-speed blender and blend until you have a smooth, vibrant green soup. Taste and adjust the seasoning to taste. Chill for 30 minutes before serving. Pour into bowls and top with a fennel frond and a drizzle of oil.

Store in an airtight glass container in the refrigerator for up to 2 days.

* * * *

BEAUTY FOOD SPOTLIGHT

With its high water content and potassium levels, the combination of the honeydew melon and cucumber in this soup maintains healthy blood pressure levels. The aloe helps promote collagen production and tissue repair, resulting in beautiful, ageless skin.

* * * *

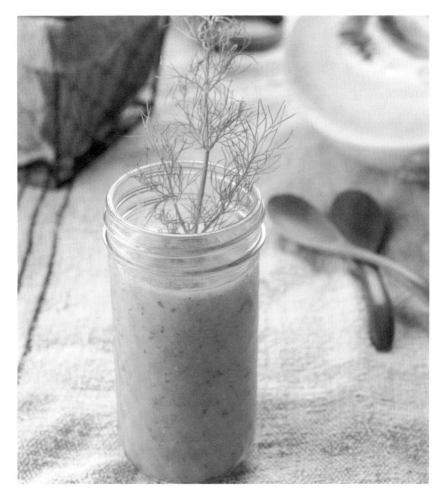

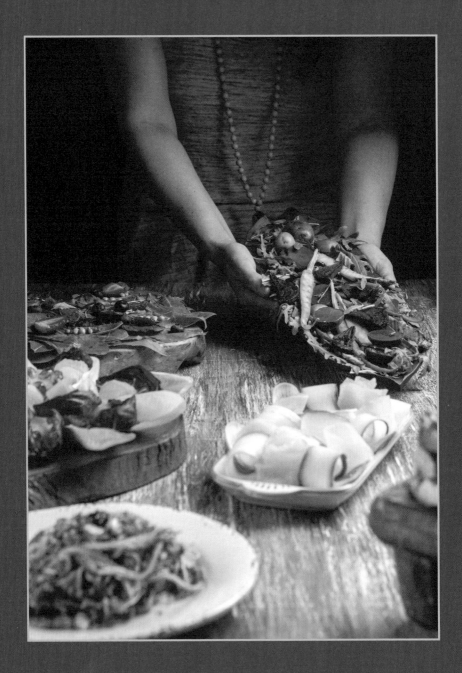

SALADS AND SLAWS

Well-Dressed and Ready for Any Occasion

Bursting with nutrients, flavor, and fiber, salads should never be relegated to the side of a plate. The salads in this chapter are a celebration of vibrant fruits and vegetables. Simple and flavorful, they are a delicious way to enjoy fresh, seasonal produce. Plus, there are six delicious superfood dressings that will have you tossing your bottled standbys in no time.

Dandelion Spring Salad

Quinoa Tabbouleh with Harissa Chickpeas

Avocado and Heirloom Tomato Tartare

Kale Thai Salad with Spicy Cashews

Rosemary Maple-Roasted Vegetable Salad

Endive, Radicchio, and Pear Salad

Celeriac, Jicama, and Apple Slaw

Cucumber Melon Ribbon Salad

6 Superfood Dressings

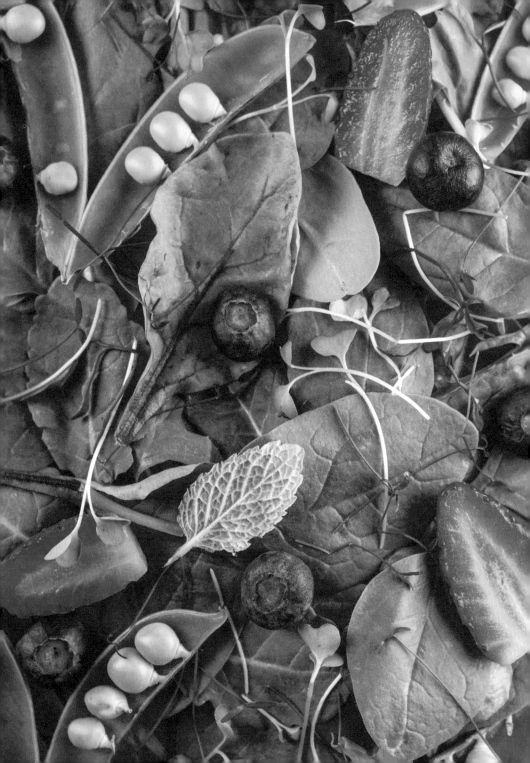

DANDELION SPRING SALAD

Light, fresh, and appealing, this lively salad screams "spring." Dandelions are great detoxifying greens, full of minerals and trace elements perfect for springtime, adding a zesty flavor to this fresh, fruit-forward salad. Toss with the Berry Beauty Elixir (page 129) and enjoy!

SERVES 4 TO 6

1 bunch dandelion greens
3 cups baby mixed greens
1 cup microgreens
1 cup sugar snap peas, deveined and split open
1 cup mixed berries
¼ cup fresh mint leaves
¼ cup fresh basil leaves
Culinary-grade flowers, for garnish (optional)
Berry Beauty Elixir (page 129)

Toss the spring vegetables together in a large bowl. When ready to serve, gently mix with the berry dressing, to avoid bruising the greens. Sprinkle with the flowers, if desired, and serve immediately.

✦ ✦ ✦ ✦

BEAUTY FOOD SPOTLIGHT

Dandelion greens are known for their powerful skin benefits and traditionally have been used as acne and eczema remedies. Dandelions' cleansing and detoxifying properties will also keep you feeling slim and trim.

✦ ✦ ✦ ✦

QUINOA TABBOULEH WITH HARISSA CHICKPEAS

Nutty quinoa pairs wonderfully with cucumbers, tomatoes, parsley, and mint and makes a great gluten-free alternative to traditional bulgur wheat in this classic, flavorful Middle Eastern salad. Quinoa is also loaded with protein, making this a satisfying main course or a hearty side, especially when served with the spiced chickpeas.

SERVES 4 TO 6

QUINOA TABBOULEH
2 cups filtered water
1 cup uncooked quinoa, rinsed well
½ cup extra-virgin olive oil
2 tablespoons fresh lemon juice
1 garlic clove, minced
1 cup diced cucumber
1 cup diced tomato
1 cup chopped fresh flat-leaf parsley
½ cup chopped fresh mint
½ cup chopped fresh basil
2 scallions, thinly sliced
Sea salt and freshly ground black pepper

✦ ✦ ✦ ✦

BEAUTY FOOD SPOTLIGHT

Quinoa, a complete-protein, gluten-free grain, is a low-glycemic complex carbohydrate that will steady your sugar and keep you full longer yet bloat free.

✦ ✦ ✦ ✦

(continued)

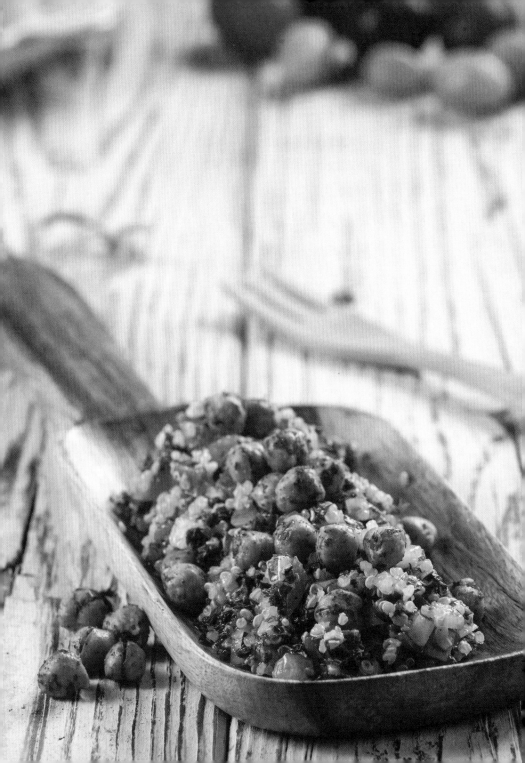

2 cups canned or cooked chickpeas, drained and rinsed
2 tablespoons olive oil
2 garlic cloves, roughly chopped
2 teaspoons harissa paste
1 teaspoon ground cumin
1 teaspoon ground coriander
1 teaspoon curry powder
Coconut yogurt, for garnish (optional)

To make the quinoa tabbouleh:

Bring in 2 cups of water to a rolling boil in a medium saucepan. Lower the heat to the lowest setting, add the quinoa, and cook, covered, for 15 minutes. Remove from the heat and let sit, covered, for 5 minutes. Fluff with a fork. Let cool.

Whisk together the olive oil, lemon juice, and garlic in a small bowl. Transfer the cooled quinoa to a large bowl along with the cucumber, tomato, parsley, mint, basil, and scallions and mix with the dressing. Adjust the seasoning to taste.

To make the harissa chickpeas:

Heat the oil in a pan over medium heat. Add the garlic and cook for 2 to 3 minutes, until fragrant. Add the harissa paste and spices and stir in the chickpeas. Mix well and cook for about 5 minutes. Taste, and adjust the seasoning if needed.

To serve, evenly distribute the quinoa tabbouleh among serving bowls and top with the harissa chickpeas. Serve with a dollop of coconut yogurt, if desired.

✦ ✦ ✦ ✦

KITCHEN NOTE

For easier digestion, try sprouting your beans, grains, nuts, and seeds to help break down their complex proteins, carbohydrates, and cellular walls. Simply soak the quinoa overnight in water, then drain and rinse it. Then cover with a towel and let sit for 6 hours. Rinse once more and allow to dry before proceeding with the recipe. No need to cook the quinoa.

✦ ✦ ✦ ✦

AVOCADO AND HEIRLOOM TOMATO TARTARE

This simplified tartare recipe makes avocado the star. Diced finely with cucumbers, cilantro, and jalapeño—and topped with juicy heirloom tomatoes—this spicy dish is festive and nourishing.

SERVES 4 TO 6

AVOCADO LAYER

2 tablespoons extra-virgin olive oil

2 tablespoons fresh lemon juice

1 tablespoon chopped fresh cilantro

½ small jalapeño pepper, minced

Sea salt and freshly ground black pepper

2 medium Hass avocados, peeled and finely diced

1 cup peeled and finely diced cucumber

TOMATO LAYER

1 tablespoon finely chopped fresh mint

1 tablespoon finely chopped fresh basil

2 tablespoons extra-virgin olive oil

2 tablespoons fresh lemon juice

Sea salt and freshly ground black pepper

2 cups finely diced heirloom tomato

4 to 6 fresh basil leaves, for garnish

(continued)

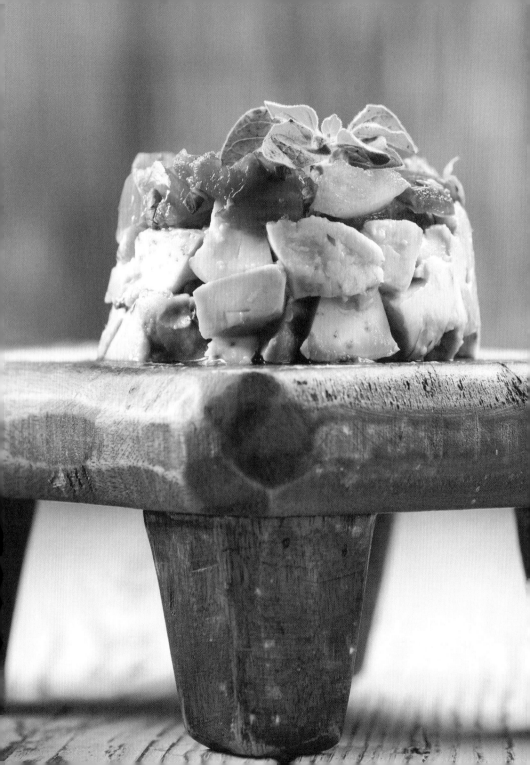

To make the avocado layer:
Stir together the olive oil, lemon juice, cilantro, and jalapeño in a medium bowl. Season with salt and black pepper. Gently fold in the avocados and cucumber.

To make the tomato layer:
Stir together the olive oil, lemon juice, mint, and basil in a medium bowl. Season with salt and pepper. Gently fold in the tomato.

Mound the avocado layer in the center of individual plates and top with a layer of the tomato mixture. Garnish each with a fresh basil leaf.

✦ ✦ ✦ ✦

BEAUTY FOOD SPOTLIGHT

Besides being some of the richest sources of monounsaturated (healthy) fats in the world, avocados are also one of the better sources of B vitamins, such as niacin, which assist your body in building and repairing DNA.

✦ ✦ ✦ ✦

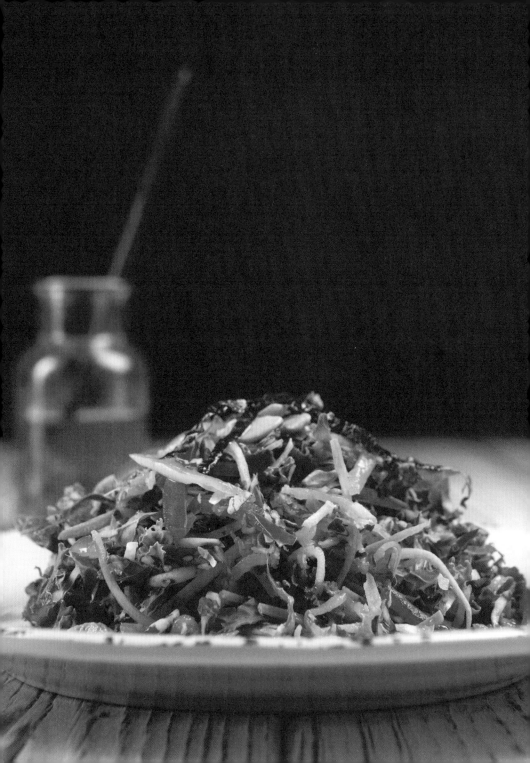

KALE THAI SALAD
WITH SPICY CASHEWS

This fun twist on the Thai salad adds kale to the mix. If you haven't made
friends with kale yet, this recipe just might change your mind.

SERVES 4 TO 6

SPICED NUTS

1½ cups raw cashews, coarsely chopped and soaked in water

¼ cup pure maple syrup

2 teaspoons chili powder

½ teaspoon sea salt

SALAD

4 cups julienned kale, thick stems removed

1 cup shredded red cabbage

1 cup julienned carrot

1 red bell pepper, seeded and julienned

1 yellow bell pepper, seeded and julienned

1 orange bell pepper, seeded and julienned

4 small sheets nori, cut into thin strips

½ cup chopped fresh cilantro

Magical Mushroom Dressing (page 126)

To make the spiced nuts:

Preheat the oven to 350°F. Line a baking sheet with parchment paper. Drain
and dry the cashews and toss them in a medium bowl with the maple syrup,

(continued)

chili powder, and salt until well coated. Spread them on the prepared baking sheet and toast for 10 to 15 minutes. Remove from the oven and let cool.

To make the salad:
Combine all the salad ingredients in a large bowl and toss with the dressing until evenly coated.

To serve, transfer to individual plates and sprinkle generously with the spiced nuts.

+ + + +

BEAUTY FOOD SPOTLIGHT

We all know kale is good for our health, but did you know that this leafy green contains 130 percent of your daily vitamin C—an essential collagen builder to keep skin firm? Kale also supports detoxification of your liver and kidneys, essential for keeping skin clear.

+ + + +

ROSEMARY MAPLE-ROASTED VEGETABLE SALAD

Tenderly roasted in rosemary and maple glazed, this vegetable medley makes a warming and grounding meal on a cool day. Mix with peppery arugula for a hardy, full-flavored experience.

SERVES 4 TO 6

Balsamic maple vinaigrette
2 tablespoons balsamic vinegar
½ cup olive oil
½ cup pure maple syrup
Juice of 1 orange

Vegetables
6 rainbow carrots, halved lengthwise
6 small beets, peeled and quartered
6 small purple potatoes, halved
2 small red onions, quartered
6 garlic cloves, unpeeled
12 asparagus stalks
4 to 6 cups or large handfuls of arugula
1 to 2 sprigs rosemary

Preheat the oven to 400°F. Line a baking sheet with parchment paper.

To make the balsamic maple vinaigrette:
Combine all the vinaigrette ingredients in a small bowl.

(continued)

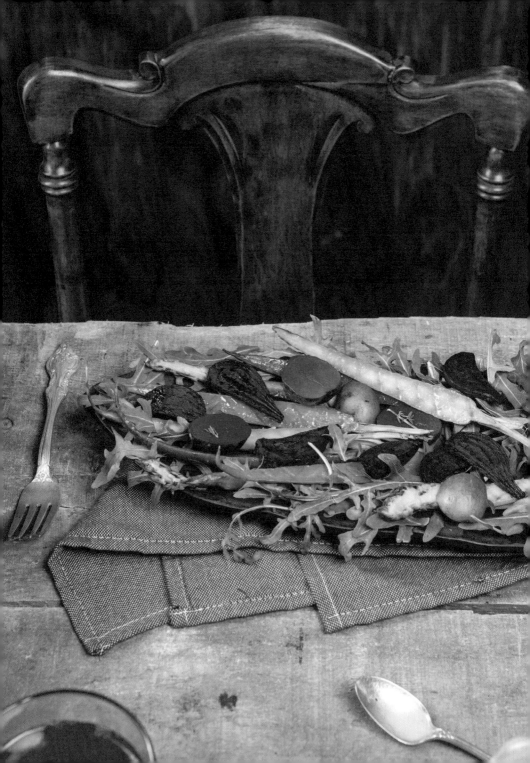

To make the vegetables:

Toss together all the vegetables in a large bowl with half of the balsamic maple vinaigrette. Transfer all the vegetables, except the asparagus, to the prepared baking sheet and roast in the oven for 20 minutes.

Remove the garlic from the baking sheet and set aside. Add the asparagus to the vegetables, tossing to combine, and return the pan to the oven for another 10 minutes, or until the vegetables have all softened.

Once fully cooked, let the roasted vegetables cool to room temperature before assembling the salad. Remove and discard the rosemary sprigs.

Meanwhile, cut the root ends of the garlic cloves, squeeze out the garlic, and mash to a paste with the side of a knife. Transfer to a large bowl and add the remaining vinaigrette. Whisk to combine.

To serve, gently toss the arugula with the balsamic maple vinaigrette in a large bowl and arrange on serving plates. Top with a generous mound of roasted vegetables.

✦ ✦ ✦ ✦

BEAUTY FOOD SPOTLIGHT

*Beets increase the body's production of glutathione, the nutrient
responsible for stimulating cell function and detoxification.
That's good news for maintaining youthful skin and protecting
the body against bruising.*

✦ ✦ ✦ ✦

ENDIVE, RADICCHIO, AND PEAR SALAD

This light, bright salad makes a refreshing starter. The distinct bitter crunch of the endive and radicchio, the sweeter crispness of the pear, and the jeweled burst of pomegranate cleanse the palate and stimulate the taste buds.

SERVES 4 TO 6

2 heads Belgian endive, cored
1 head red radicchio, quartered and cored
2 Asian pears, quartered, cored, and thinly sliced
½ cup pomegranate arils
½ cup fresh lemon juice
½ cup warm walnut oil
½ cup walnuts, toasted and roughly chopped

Place the endive and radicchio in a shallow serving bowl. Top with the pear slices and pomegranate. Stir together the lemon juice and warm walnut oil in a small bowl and drizzle on top of the salad. Top with the toasted walnuts.

✦ ✦ ✦ ✦

KITCHEN NOTE

To toast the walnuts, spread them out in a dry skillet and cook for about a minute on medium heat, moving the skillet back and forth. Promptly remove the nuts from the pan to stop the cooking.

✦ ✦ ✦ ✦

BEAUTY FOOD SPOTLIGHT

The powerful combination of vitamins A, C, and K in radicchio offers cooling, toning beauty benefits that can help reduce dark circles under the eyes.

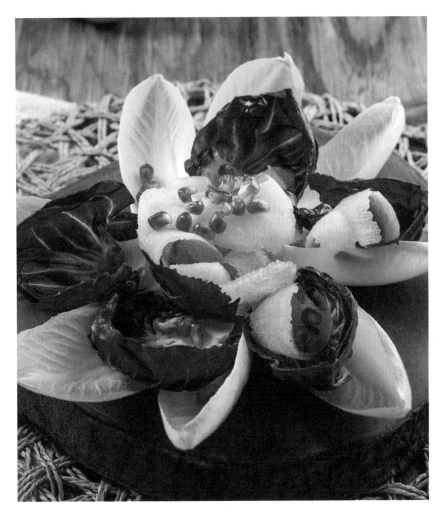

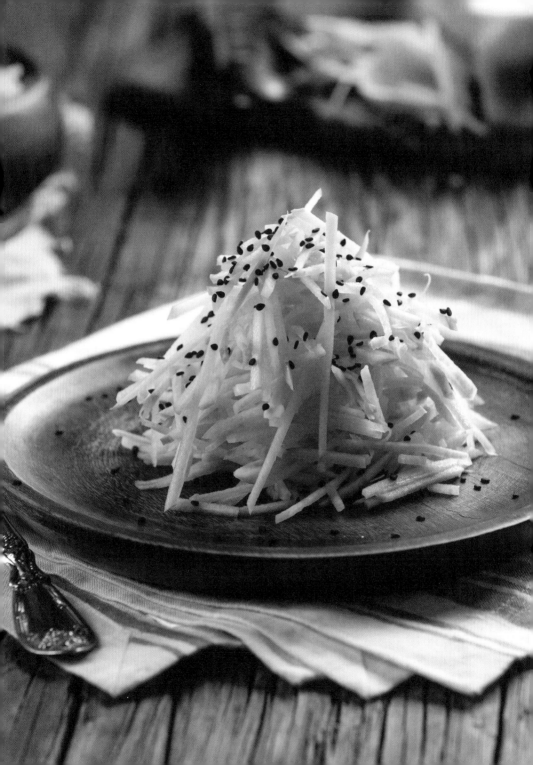

CELERIAC, JICAMA, AND APPLE SLAW

This nutrient-dense play on coleslaw combines celeriac, jicama, and apple for a medley of flavors. Toss this sweet and tangy slaw with the Sesame Scallion Dressing (page 125) for a tasty crunch.

SERVES 4 TO 6

2 cups trimmed, peeled, and julienned celeriac
2 cups cored and julienned Granny Smith apple
2 cups julienned jicama
Sesame Scallion Dressing (page 125)

Combine the celeriac, apple, and jicama in a large bowl and toss with the dressing until evenly coated. Divide among serving bowls.

✦ ✦ ✦ ✦

BEAUTY FOOD SPOTLIGHT

Celeriac is a highly alkalizing food that supports the healthy pH balance in our skin. Also high in copper, phosphorus, and vitamin K, celeriac promotes strong bones and healthy teeth.

✦ ✦ ✦ ✦

CUCUMBER MELON RIBBON SALAD

This lovely salad combines refreshing cucumber with sweet, delicate honeydew and crisp, peppery radish. A drizzle of the sunshine dressing is all you need to let this salad shine.

SERVES 4 TO 6

1 medium honeydew melon
2 medium English cucumbers
4 to 6 watermelon radishes

Sᴜɴꜱʜɪɴᴇ ᴅʀᴇꜱꜱɪɴɢ
2 tablespoons olive oil
1 teaspoon freshly grated citrus zest
Juice of 1 orange
Juice of 1 lemon
¼ cup chopped fresh mint
Sea salt and freshly ground black pepper
2 tablespoons toasted nuts and/or seeds of your liking

Remove the rind and seeds from the honeydew and cut the melon lengthwise into strips. Slice off the ends of the cucumbers and radishes. Using a vegetable peeler, shave the honeydew and cucumber into ribbons and transfer them to a bowl. For the radishes, thinly slice with a mandoline or knife and add them to the cucumbers and melon.

To make the dressing:

Whisk together the oil, citrus zest, and citrus juice in a small bowl. Add the mint and drizzle over the salad. Toss to combine. Taste and adjust the seasoning to taste. Transfer to a serving plate and sprinkle with the toasted nuts and seeds.

✦ ✦ ✦ ✦

BEAUTY FOOD SPOTLIGHT

Originally cultivated in China, the colorful watermelon radish is a nutritious root vegetable with a high phytochemical profile, including zeaxanthin, lutein, and beta-carotene, which assist your body in rebuilding tissues and blood vessels, including strong, beautiful nails. These crisp, peppery veggies also help ease digestion and reduce water retention, to keep that tummy flat.

✦ ✦ ✦ ✦

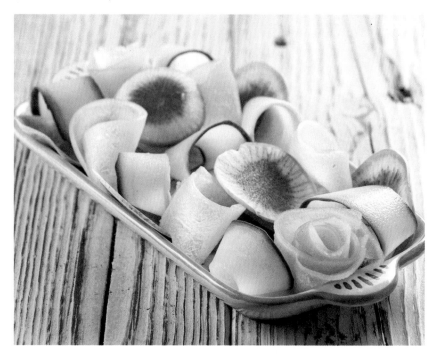

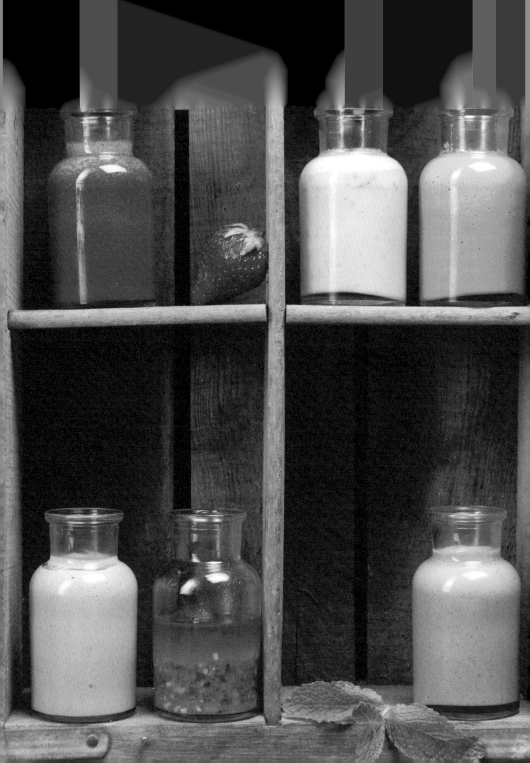

6 SUPERFOOD DRESSINGS

Preparing your own salad dressings is one beauty skill worth developing.

Don't skip the dressing to cut down on calories! Healthy fat is essential for your body to absorb the fat-soluble vitamins, such as A, E, and K, that you find in fresh veggies. Beyond containing healthy fats, the following salad dressings are brimming with beauty-boosting extras, such as fresh herbs, nuts and seeds, antioxidant-rich spices, anti-inflammatory roots, and even fermented sauces and vinegars.

SESAME SCALLION

This circulation-boosting dressing fires up digestion and immunity. Plus, the gingerol in ginger suppresses our cell-aging mechanism, keeping our skin most youthful.

MAKES 1½ CUPS

1 tablespoon minced fresh ginger

1 tablespoon minced scallions

¼ cup umeboshi plum vinegar

¼ cup fresh lemon juice

¼ cup tamari (or coconut aminos, for a soy-free option)

½ cup sesame oil

2 tablespoons black sesame seeds

Sea salt and freshly ground black pepper

Place all the ingredients, except the sesame seeds, in a blender and process until smooth. Mix in the sesame seeds and transfer to an airtight glass bottle. Store in the refrigerator for up to 1 week.

(continued)

CARROT GINGER

The carrot, ginger, turmeric, and raw apple cider vinegar in this lovely dressing support our digestion, keeping our tummy flat.

MAKES 1½ CUPS

1 cup roughly chopped carrot
1 (2-inch) piece fresh ginger, roughly chopped
1 (1-inch) piece fresh turmeric, roughly chopped
2 tablespoons tamari (or coconut aminos, for a soy-free option)
¼ cup olive oil
¼ cup fresh orange juice
2 tablespoons raw apple cider vinegar
Sea salt and freshly ground black pepper

Place all the ingredients, including salt and pepper to taste, in a blender and blend until smooth. Transfer to an airtight glass bottle. Store in the refrigerator for up to 1 week.

MAGICAL MUSHROOM

Get your antiaging fix by elevating your regular tahini dressing with a spoonful of adaptogenic mushroom powder.

MAKES 1½ CUPS

½ cup sesame oil
½ cup fresh lemon juice
¼ cup tahini
2 garlic cloves, minced
2 teaspoons medicinal mushroom powder
Sea salt and freshly ground black pepper

Whisk together all the ingredients, including salt and pepper to taste, in a bowl. Transfer to an airtight glass bottle. Store in the refrigerator for up to 1 week.

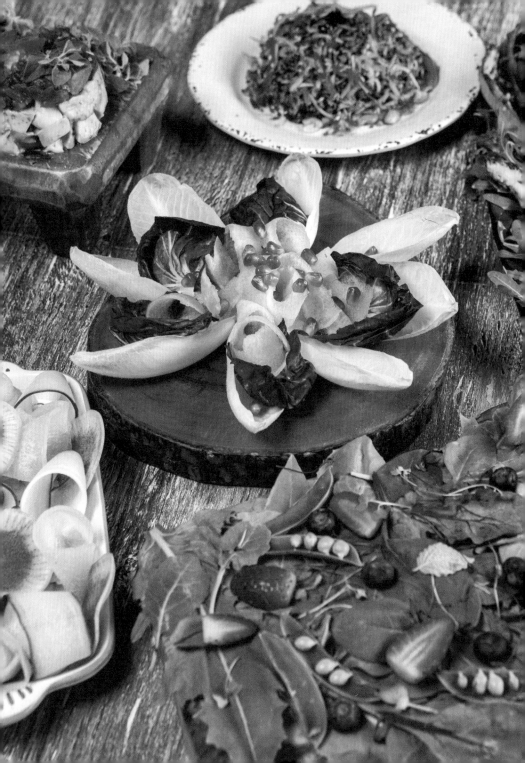

GREEN GODDESS

Fresh herbs are brimming with beauty benefits. Use skin-loving mint and basil in this dressing, or substitute for fresh dill and parsley.

MAKES 2 CUPS

1 avocado
¼ cup fresh basil
¼ cup fresh mint
¼ cup spinach, rinsed
2 garlic cloves
½ cup hemp oil
¼ cup fresh lemon juice
½ teaspoon spirulina (optional)
2 tablespoons hemp seeds (optional)
Filtered water

Place all the ingredients in a blender and blend until smooth and creamy, adding filtered water 1 tablespoon at a time until your desired consistency is achieved. Transfer to an airtight glass bottle. Store in the refrigerator for up to 2 days.

BERRY BEAUTY ELIXIR

Find that extra dose of anthocyanins from the beet and berries for optimal skin protection in this crimson elixir.

MAKES 2 CUPS

½ cup mixed berries
¼ cup beet juice
½ cup sunflower oil
¼ cup fresh lemon juice
¼ cup pure maple syrup
1 tablespoon Dijon mustard

Place all the ingredients in a blender and blend until smooth. Transfer to an airtight glass bottle. Store in the refrigerator for up to 1 week.

TROPICAL CITRUS

All the vitamin C love you need to nurture strong, beautiful hair and nails.

MAKES 2 CUPS

1 cup roughly chopped pineapple
¼ roughly chopped fresh cilantro
½ cup fresh orange juice
¼ cup fresh lime juice
¼ cup olive oil

Place all the ingredients in a blender and blend until smooth. Transfer to an airtight glass bottle. Store in the refrigerator for up to 1 week.

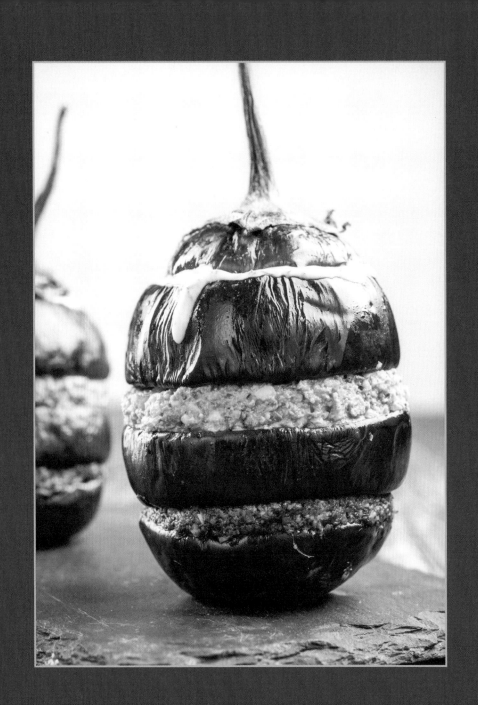

ENTRÉES AND MAINS

Warm and Hearty Dishes

The dishes in this section have the chew factor we all crave. Food needs to taste good, regardless of our dietary preferences, and the following recipes deliver with every bite. Nourishing, strengthening, and beautifying, these warm meals will leave you full, satisfied, and supported.

Eggplant Lasagne

Rainbow Noodles with Marinara and Lentil Balls

Saffron Cauli-Rice with Currants and Pine Nuts in Baked Tomatoes

Wild Mushroom Spinach Tarts

Pomegranate-Glazed Pumpkin Ravioli with Almond Thyme Pâté

Artichoke Cakes with Dill Yogurt

Jackfruit Carnitas Tacos

Smoky Portobello Steak with Chimichurri Sauce

EGGPLANT LASAGNE

This is not your mama's lasagne, but no less hearty and satisfying. Full of healthful omega-3 fatty acids and protein, this versatile dish can be put together in a number of ways, depending on the type of eggplant you decide on. You can go the more traditional way by slicing up long strips of eggplant to put together, or my favorite for parties, the interactive method, where you bake small individual eggplants for each dinner guest and have them build their own! See the result on page 130.

SERVES 4 TO 6

2 medium or 6 small eggplants

ALMOND RICOTTA

2 cups almonds, blanched and soaked overnight in water, then drained
2 tablespoons fresh lemon juice
6 tablespoons filtered water, used as needed
Sea salt
Freshly ground black pepper

WALNUT BOLOGNESE

2 cups walnuts
1 teaspoon dried thyme
1 teaspoon dried rosemary
1 teaspoon dried sage
Sea salt and freshly ground black pepper
1 cup Marinara Sauce (page 136)
Nettle and Hemp Seed Pesto (page 65)

Slice the eggplants lengthwise and set aside.

To make the almond ricotta:
Place all the ricotta ingredients in your food processor or blender and process until smooth and thick, adding as little water as possible. Set aside.

To make the walnut Bolognese:
Place all the Bolognese ingredients, except the marinara, in your food processor or blender and blend, keeping the mixture thick and chunky. Transfer to a bowl and stir in the marinara sauce. Set aside.

Preheat the oven to 375°F. Layer the eggplant, Bolognese, pesto, and ricotta cheese in a baking pan, alternating as you go, reserving any extra Bolognese and ricotta for serving. Brush the tops and sides of the eggplant with olive oil. Add ½ cup of warm water to the bottom of the pan in between the eggplants and bake for 30 to 40 minutes, until the eggplant has softened. Remove from the oven and let cool for 5 minutes.

Serve warm with extra servings of Bolognese and ricotta.

✦ ✦ ✦ ✦

BEAUTY FOOD SPOTLIGHT

The phenolic compound in eggplants, the same compound that gives this vegetable their unique color, also helps build stronger bones and mineral bone density. They are powerful sources of phytonutrients that help boost cognitive activity. They also defend against free radical activity and keep your body and brain safe from toxins and diseases.

✦ ✦ ✦ ✦

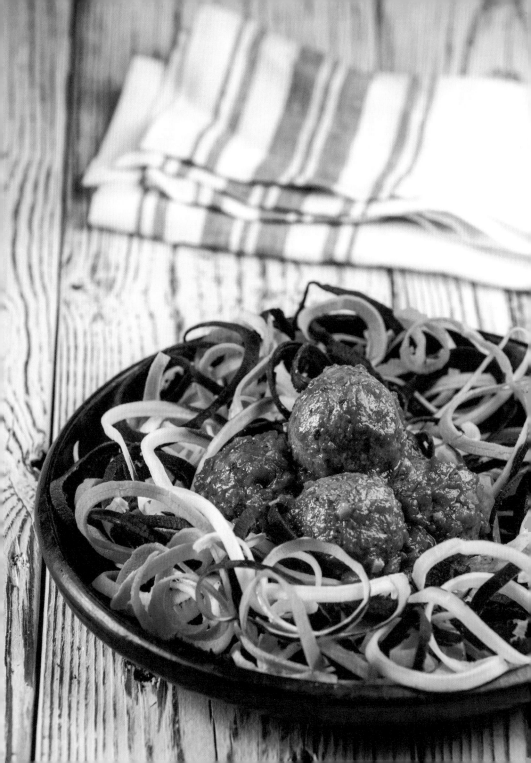

RAINBOW NOODLES WITH MARINARA AND LENTIL BALLS

Tender and savory, these protein-rich meatballs, high in folate, support cell building and repair for enviable hair, skin, and nails. Perfect atop a vibrant bowl of nutritious vegetable noodles and zesty homemade marinara sauce.

SERVES 4

Lentil balls

Olive oil

½ cup minced white onion

3 garlic cloves, minced

½ cup walnuts

1 cup cooked and cooled yellow lentils

½ cup diced dried apricots

1 teaspoon dried basil

1 teaspoon dried oregano

1 tablespoon dried parsley

¼ cup nutritional yeast (optional)

Sea salt and freshly ground black pepper

2 tablespoons flaxseed meal (optional)

(continued)

1 zucchini

1 carrot

1 parsnip

1 beet

½ cup olive oil

4 medium garlic cloves

1 teaspoon dried herbs (optional)

MARINARA SAUCE

1 red onion, diced

2 garlic cloves, peeled and minced

1 cup chopped sun-dried tomatoes, soaked for 1 hour in water

1 cup diced fresh tomato

½ cup olive oil

Juice of ½ lemon

2 teaspoons Italian seasoning

Make the lentil balls:

Preheat the oven to 375°F. Line a baking sheet with parchment paper.

Heat the oil in a skillet over medium heat. Add the onion and garlic and sauté for 2 to 3 minutes. Remove from the heat. Place the walnuts in a food processor and pulse to break them into small chunks. Add the cooked lentils, sautéed onion mixture, apricots, herbs, nutritional yeast, if using, and salt and pepper to taste. Pulse to combine, leaving a little texture.

If the mixture is too wet, add flaxseed meal 1 teaspoon at a time until you can form balls with your hands. Using a tablespoon, scoop out the mixture and carefully form into 1½-inch balls. Arrange on baking sheet.

Bake for 30 minutes, turning the balls at the 15-minute point. Remove from the oven and let cool slightly—they will firm up the longer they are cooled.

Make the noodles:

Cut the veggies lengthwise into thin strips, using a mandoline or spiral slicer, then mix together in a bowl and set aside. Pour the olive oil into a small sauté pan and use a garlic press to crush the garlic cloves directly into the oil. Add your favorite herbs or spices. Gently heat the oil over medium-low heat, stirring often, until the garlic is crispy and golden brown and the aromatics release their fragrance, 3 to 5 minutes. Remove from the heat immediately and transfer to a bowl to cool. Strain the oil.

Use 1 tablespoon of the infused oil to coat the vegetable noodles. Toss gently to combine. Allow to infuse for 5 minutes.

The flavored oil can be stored in an airtight container, refrigerated, for up to 2 weeks.

Make the marinara sauce:

Blend all the ingredients until smooth.

To serve, divide the noodles among individual plates, add a serving of lentil balls and top with fresh marinara sauce. Sprinkle with Seed Parmesan (page 200).

This dish is best when fresh, although leftovers keep in the freezer up to 1 month. Reheat in a 350°F oven until warmed through.

SAFFRON CAULI-RICE WITH CURRANTS AND PINE NUTS IN BAKED TOMATOES

Stuffed with saffron-infused cauliflower rice, plump currants, sweet apricots, and savory pine nuts, these baked tomatoes keep your electrolytes in balance and your skin radiantly hydrated.

SERVES 6

6 large tomatoes
1 tablespoon pine nuts
1 medium (2-pound) cauliflower
2 tablespoons olive oil, plus more for brushing
½ cup chopped onion
¼ cup finely chopped dried apricots
1 tablespoon dried currants
1 teaspoon ground cumin
1 teaspoon ground cinnamon
½ teaspoon saffron threads
Sea salt and freshly ground black pepper
1 tablespoon finely chopped fresh mint, for garnish

Preheat the oven to 375°F.

Slice the top of each tomato to make small lids. Scoop out the insides and save 1 cup. Chop the flesh and set aside.

Toast the pine nuts in a pan over medium heat for 2 to 3 minutes, until golden.

(continued)

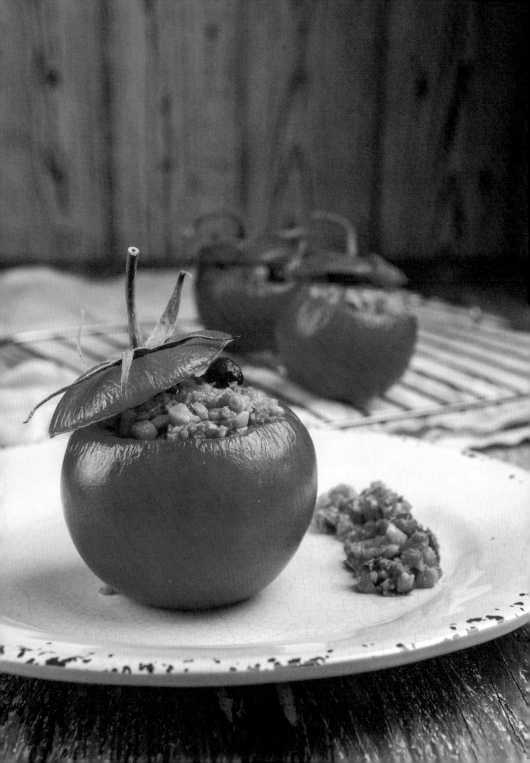

Trim the cauliflower, cutting away the stems. Break up the florets into a food processor and pulse until the mixture resembles rice. Use 2 cups of the rice for this recipe.

Heat the oil in a large skillet over medium-high heat. Add the onion and sauté for 2 to 3 minutes. Add the reserved tomato flesh and cauliflower rice; stir to combine.

Add the apricots, currants, pine nuts, cumin, cinnamon, saffron, and salt and pepper to taste and continue to cook, stirring frequently, until the cauliflower has softened, 3 to 5 minutes. Remove from the heat.

Allow to cool for about 10 minutes before filling the tomatoes. Fill the tomatoes to the top with the cauli-rice filling and cover them with their respective lids.

Place the stuffed tomatoes in a baking pan. Brush the tops and sides of the tomatoes with olive oil. Add ½ cup of warm water to the bottom of the pan in between the stuffed tomatoes and bake for 30 minutes.

Remove from the oven and let cool for 5 minutes.

Serve warm with a generous sprinkle of fresh mint.

✦ ✦ ✦ ✦

BEAUTY FOOD SPOTLIGHT

The exotic spice saffron is highly prized for its color, flavor, and medicinal properties. The dried stigma of the crocus flower, it contains high concentrations of nutrients that stimulate the immune system's production of white blood cells, the body's first line of defense against illness, and that are also crucial to the production of collagen, essential for healthy hair, pretty nails, and glowing skin.

✦ ✦ ✦ ✦

WILD MUSHROOM SPINACH TARTS

These enchanting crustless tartlets made with creamy cashews, savory mushrooms, and a vibrant pop of spinach are rich in iron and selenium, a trace mineral that protects our skin's elasticity.

SERVES 4

MARINATED MUSHROOMS
⅓ cup olive oil
⅓ cup balsamic vinegar
2 garlic cloves, minced
2 cups chopped mixed wild mushrooms

FILLING
2 cups raw cashews, soaked in water overnight, then drained
Juice of ½ lemon
1 garlic clove, chopped
3 tablespoons chopped shallot
Sea salt
1 cup marinated mushrooms, drained
1 cup spinach, rinsed and chopped
Fresh herbs, for serving

Make the marinated mushrooms:
Whisk together the olive oil, balsamic vinegar, and garlic. Pour over the mushrooms, cover, and let marinate for 1 hour in the refrigerator.

(continued)

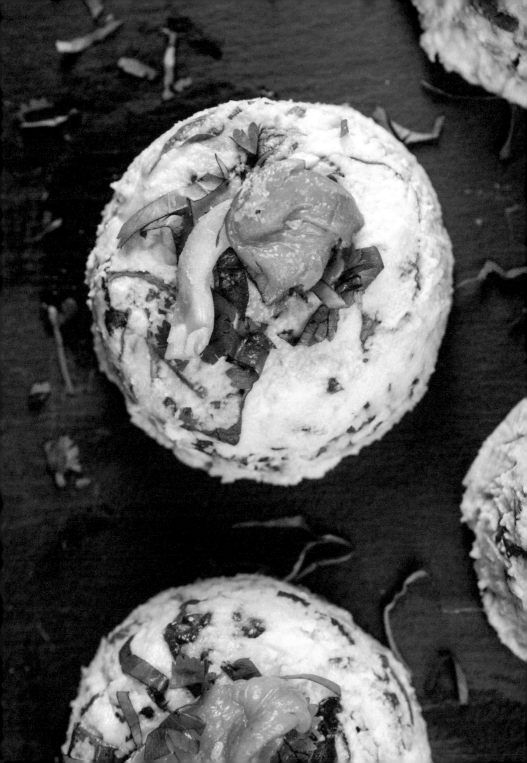

Make the filling:

Place the soaked cashews in a food processor or blender along with the lemon juice, garlic, shallot, and salt. Process to a thick mixture, then spoon into a medium bowl. Add the drained marinated mushrooms and spinach and mix to combine.

Line a 6-well muffin tin with plastic wrap and pack tightly with the mixture.

Cover and refrigerate for at least 2 hours.

Carefully remove the tarts from their molds. To serve, sprinkle with fresh herbs.

+ + + +

BEAUTY FOOD SPOTLIGHT

Mushrooms are great sources of selenium, copper, niacin, potassium, and phosphorous. They also provide protein, vitamin C, and iron. Because mushroom cell walls are indigestible unless exposed to heat, you should cook mushrooms to get their maximum nutritional benefits.

+ + + +

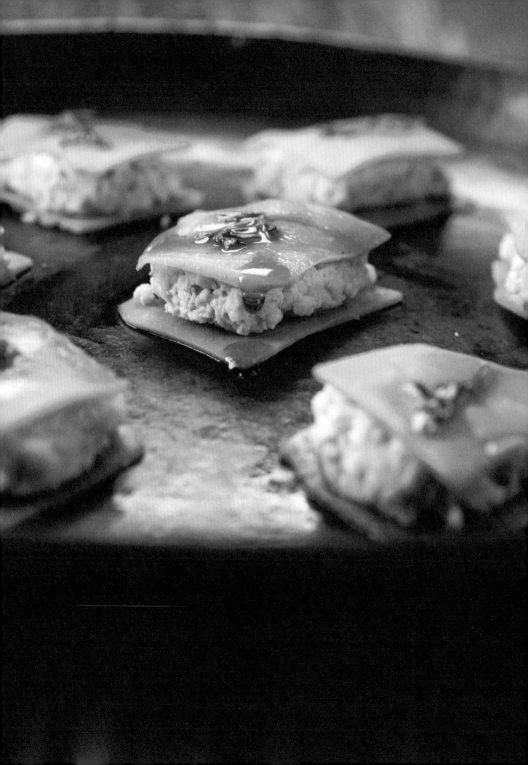

POMEGRANATE-GLAZED PUMPKIN RAVIOLI WITH ALMOND THYME PÂTÉ

I love the delicate flavors in this deconstructed ravioli dish. The sweetly marinated pumpkin slices are filled with a creamy almond thyme pâté and topped with a simple yet intoxicating pomegranate glaze.

SERVES 4

ALMOND THYME PÂTÉ

1 cup almonds, blanched and soaked overnight in water, then drained

2 tablespoons fresh lemon juice

2 garlic cloves

1 tablespoon fresh thyme leaves

Sea salt

POMEGRANATE GLAZE

1 cup pomegranate juice

1 tablespoon pure maple syrup

1 tablespoon fresh lemon juice

(continued)

PUMPKIN RAVIOLI
1 medium (2-pound) sugar pumpkin
1 teaspoon fresh thyme leaves, plus more for serving
3 tablespoons grapeseed oil
2 tablespoons fresh orange juice
Sea salt
Freshly ground black pepper

To make the pâté:
Place all the pâté ingredients in a food processor or a blender and process until smooth and thick. Adjust the salt to taste and set aside.

To make the glaze:
Combine all the glaze ingredients in a small saucepan and bring to a boil. Lower the heat to a simmer and cook for 15 minutes. Set aside.

To make the pumpkin ravioli:
Using a mandoline, slice the pumpkin very thinly, then use a knife to cut the slices into squares of roughly the same size. You should have about 16 slices (for 8 ravioli) per serving. To make the marinade: Combine the pumpkin slices, thyme, olive oil, orange juice, and a generous pinch of sea salt in a medium bowl. Toss to coat. Let marinate for 15 minutes.

Arrange half of the pumpkin slices flat on serving plates. Place 1 teaspoon of the pâté on each slice and top with a reserved pumpkin slice. Top the ravioli with pomegranate glaze and sauce each plate with the remaining glaze. Sprinkle with pepper and extra thyme.

✦ ✦ ✦ ✦

BEAUTY FOOD SPOTLIGHT

Pumpkin's brilliant orange coloring comes from its ample supply of beta-carotene, which is converted to vitamin A in the body. Vitamin A is essential for beautiful nails, bones, and teeth and helps protect us from the sun's UV rays.

✦ ✦ ✦ ✦

ARTICHOKE CAKES WITH DILL YOGURT

These delicious cakes are light, tasty, and so similar in look and texture to traditional crab cakes, you might have a hard time convincing your guests they're made of artichokes.

MAKES 6 TO 8 CAKES

DILL YOGURT
½ cup Cashew Yogurt (page 201)
1 tablespoon finely chopped fresh dill
Sea salt and freshly ground black pepper

CAKES
2 cups marinated artichoke hearts, drained (reserve 6 tablespoons of the marinade)
2 tablespoons flaxseed meal, plus more if needed
¼ cup finely chopped shallot
½ cup finely chopped celery
1 teaspoon fresh lemon juice
1 tablespoon Old Bay Seasoning
Sea salt and freshly ground black pepper
Olive oil, for cooking

To make the dill yogurt:
Stir together all the sauce ingredients, including salt and pepper to taste, in a small bowl until well combined. Refrigerate until ready to serve.

(continued)

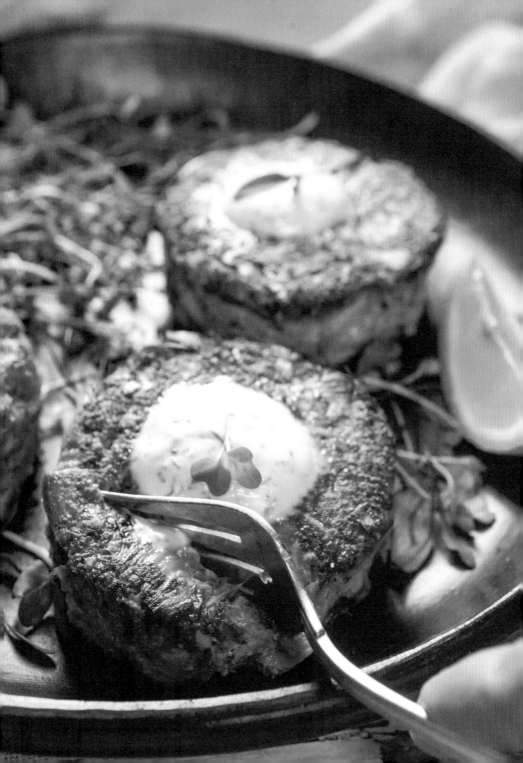

To make the cakes:

Place the reserved artichoke liquid in a small bowl and stir in the 2 tablespoons of flaxseed meal. Let sit for 5 minutes.

Chop the artichoke hearts and transfer to a large bowl along with the shallot, celery, flaxseed mixture, lemon, Old Bay Seasoning, and salt and pepper to taste. Combine with a fork. You should be able to use your hands to form 2½-inch-thick patties. If the mixture is too wet, add additional flaxseed meal, 1 teaspoon at a time, to help form the patties. Refrigerate for 30 minutes.

To panfry:

Heat the oil in a large, nonstick skillet. When the oil is hot, add the patties. Cook for 4 to 5 minutes on each side, until browned.

To bake:

Preheat the oven to 350°F while the patties chill. Line a baking sheet with parchment paper.

Place the patties on the prepared baking sheet and bake for 15 minutes. Then, using a spatula, gently flip each patty and return the baking sheet to the oven for another 15 minutes, or until the patties are firm and golden.

Remove from the oven and let cool slightly. Serve with a generous dollop of dill yogurt sauce.

Store in an airtight glass container in the refrigerator for up to 3 days.

+ + + +

BEAUTY FOOD SPOTLIGHT

The humble artichoke is packed with a number of vital antioxidants and phytonutrients, such as quercetin, rutin, gallic acid, and cynarin, which your body requires to combat free radicals and to slow the aging process. The artichoke also helps detox your body by nourishing the digestive tract and ensuring you always fit in your skinny jeans.

+ + + +

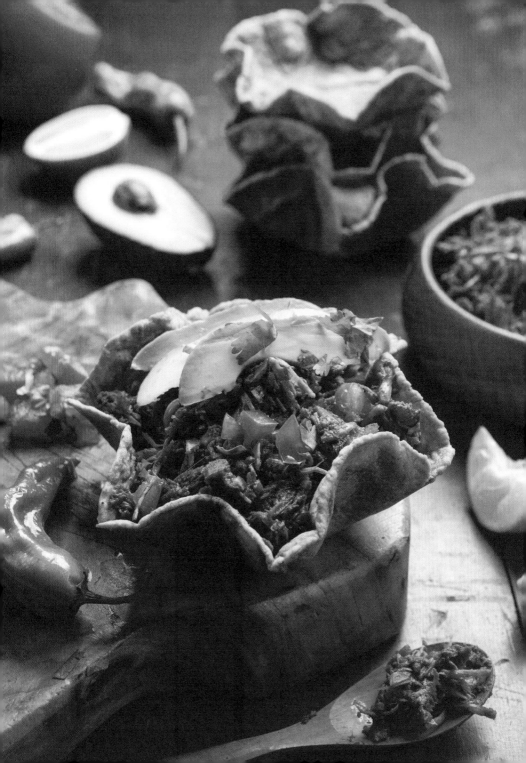

JACKFRUIT CARNITAS TACOS

Carnitas taco lovers, rejoice! This jackfruit re-creation of the original pulled pork taco is quite remarkable. The jackfruit shreds and falls apart just like its meaty counterpart, while its neutral taste makes it the perfect ingredient to marinate.

SERVES 4 TO 6

JACKFRUIT CARNITAS

2 tablespoons olive oil

1 teaspoon paprika

1 teaspoon chili powder

1 tablespoon tamari (or coconut aminos, for a soy-free option)

1 tablespoon pure maple syrup

1 medium onion, minced

4 garlic cloves, minced

1 (20-ounce) can jackfruit in water, drained and rinsed well

1 cup Vegetable Beauty Broth (page 78)

1 chipotle pepper in adobo sauce, finely chopped

✦ ✦ ✦ ✦

BEAUTY FOOD SPOTLIGHT

Jackfruit is a delicious fruit packed with powerful antiulcerative, antiseptic, and anti-inflammatory properties. The largest tree-borne fruit in the world, jackfruit fulfills the iron needs in the body, promoting proper blood circulation and preventing anemia. It is also known to inhibit the degeneration of cells, to help maintain younger, suppler, and more glowing skin.

✦ ✦ ✦ ✦

(continued)

SPINACH TORTILLAS
4 cups spinach, rinsed
¼ cup water, plus more if needed
2 tablespoons olive oil
1 cup tapioca flour
Sea salt
Fresh lime juice, for serving

To make the jackfruit carnitas:
Place the olive oil, paprika, chili powder, tamari, maple syrup, onion, and garlic in a large bowl and mix well. Add the jackfruit and allow to marinate for 2 hours.

Heat a large skillet over medium heat. Add the marinated jackfruit and its marinade, vegetable broth, and chipotle pepper. Mix well and bring to a boil. Lower the heat to low and simmer, covered, stirring occasionally.

After 20 minutes, uncover the pan and use a fork to break up the jackfruit. Continue to cook for another 15 minutes, or until the sauce is absorbed, stirring often to break up the larger pieces of jackfruit.

To make the spinach tortillas:
Place the spinach and the ¼ cup of water in a large pan and simmer over low heat for 3 minutes, or until the spinach wilts. Transfer the spinach and its cooking water to a food processor or blender, add the oil, and process until smooth. Let cool.

Whisk together the tapioca flour and salt in a large bowl. Stir in the spinach mixture and knead by hand into a dough until smooth and soft. If the dough appears too dry or sticky, sprinkle with a tablespoon of water. Divide the dough into six equal-size balls, cover, and place in the refrigerator for 20 minutes. Place a ball of dough between two pieces of parchment paper and roll out to make a 6- to 8-inch tortilla. Heat a dry nonstick pan over low heat and place the tortilla in the hot pan for 4 minutes. Flip and cook the tortilla for another 4 minutes. Remove and repeat to make the remaining tortillas.

To serve, divide the chipotle jackfruit among the tortilla shells, squeeze lime juice on top, and garnish with salsa, vegan sour cream, or avocado slices.

SMOKY PORTOBELLO STEAK WITH CHIMICHURRI SAUCE

Glazed and grilled to perfection, the portobello in this simple recipe is transformed into a hardy, smoky steak. Top it with a generous helping of chimichurri, the fresh, spicy grilling sauce from Argentina.

SERVES 4

CHIMICHURRI SAUCE
¾ cup finely chopped fresh parsley
¼ cup finely chopped fresh cilantro
2 tablespoons finely chopped fresh mint
4 garlic cloves, minced
1 small white onion, minced
1 tablespoon dried oregano
1 teaspoon red pepper flakes
½ cup olive oil
Juice of 1 lime
Sea salt and freshly ground black pepper

PORTOBELLO STEAKS AND MUSHROOM GLAZE
1 teaspoon Lapsang Souchong tea leaves or liquid smoke
1 teaspoon umeboshi plum vinegar
¼ cup olive oil
Sea salt and freshly ground black pepper
4 large portobello mushroom caps, cleaned
Fresh greens, for serving

(continued)

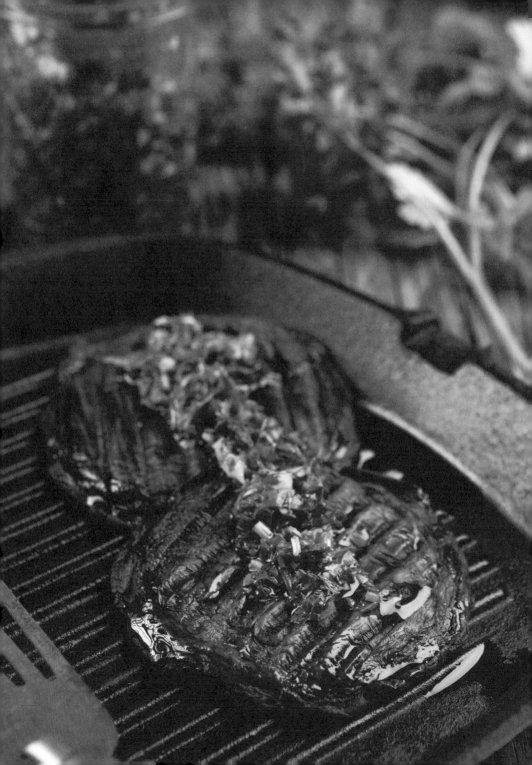

To make the chimichurri: sauce:
Place all the sauce ingredients, including salt and black pepper to taste, in a food processor or blender and process until smooth. Adjust the seasoning, if necessary. Transfer the sauce to a bowl and set aside for at least 20 minutes.

To make the mushroom glaze:
Place all the ingredients, including salt and pepper to taste, in a food processor or blender and process until smooth. Adjust the seasoning, if necessary.

Transfer the sauce to a bowl and brush both sides of each mushroom thoroughly with the glaze.

Heat a grill or a large skillet over medium heat and place a mushroom inside, ribbed side up. Pour any remaining marinade over the mushroom. Cook for 3 to 4 minutes on each side. Cook the remaining mushrooms in the same way.

To serve, place each portobello steak on a bed of fresh greens and top with a generous helping of chimichurri sauce.

✦ ✦ ✦ ✦

BEAUTY FOOD SPOTLIGHT

Harvested, rolled, oxidized, and dried over pinewood fires, Lapsang Souchong Chinese black tea has an intense, smoky taste. Adding the tea to the marinade will impart its lovely smokiness to the mushrooms. Lapsang Souchong contains powerful antioxidants, such as catechins and polyphenols, which aid in preventing free radicals in our body. This smoky tea can also lower blood pressure and manage blood sugar.

✦ ✦ ✦ ✦

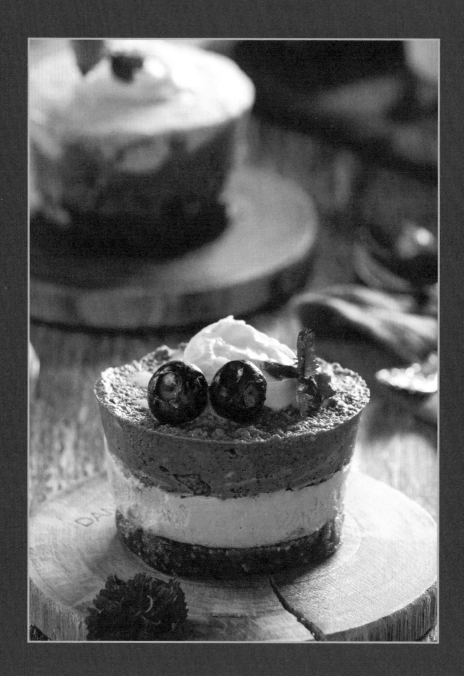

SWEET ENDINGS

Desserts and Sweet Treats

What if the sweet, indulgent rewards we crave weren't such a guilty pleasure? What if, instead, we had sweets with benefits? Packed with antioxidants, minerals, and phytochemicals—without any refined sugars or unhealthy starches—the following desserts are truly worth celebrating. So, grab a friend and a spoon and dig in!

Blueberry Maqui Cheesecake

Raw Lavender Lemon Cookies

Raw Matcha Key Lime Cupcakes

Golden Milk Ice-Cream Brownie Sandwiches

Carrot Cake Donuts with Citrus Cream Cheese Frosting

Mille Crepe Cake with Salted Crème Caramel

BLUEBERRY MAQUI CHEESECAKE

A healthy nondairy version of cheesecake? Absolutely! You'll love this completely raw recipe for the creamiest, berry cashew cheese filling with a dense, chewy, chocolatey crust made of walnuts, coconuts, dates, and raw cacao. Pictured on page 156.

SERVES 10 TO 12

CRUST
1 cup dates, pitted
½ cup unsweetened shredded coconut
1 cup walnuts
1 tablespoon raw cacao powder
Sea salt

FILLING
2 cups raw cashews, soaked in water overnight, then drained
½ cup fresh lemon juice
½ cup coconut oil
½ cup pure maple syrup
1 teaspoon pure vanilla extract
Water, as needed

BLUEBERRY MAQUI LAYER
¼ cup blueberries
2 teaspoons maqui powder (optional)

To make the crust:
Place the dates, coconut, walnuts, cacao powder, and salt in a food processor or blender and process to a coarse meal. Transfer the mixture to a springform pan or individual tart shells and press down to form the crust. Place in the freezer to chill.

To make the filling:
Place the filling ingredients in a high-speed blender and blend. Add as little water as necessary to facilitate blending. Pour half of the mixture on top of your crust and place in the freezer for 1 hour. Reserve the rest of the filling in the blender to make the blueberry maqui layer.

To make the blueberry maqui layer:
Add the blueberries and maqui powder, if using, to the reserved filling in the blender and blend once more.

Pour the maqui layer on top of the frozen cheesecake and freeze overnight. Let the cheesecake sit at room temperature for 15 minutes before serving.

✦ ✦ ✦ ✦

BEAUTY FOOD SPOTLIGHT

Although a completely optional ingredient in this cheesecake, the beautiful purple maqui berry contains antioxidant compounds that boost skin's connective tissue, your first defense against wrinkles.

✦ ✦ ✦ ✦

RAW LAVENDER LEMON COOKIES

Cookies with benefits! These delicately fragrant cookies are so simple to make and delightfully full of natural ingredients. The perfect treat to enjoy with a cup of tea.

MAKES 2 DOZEN

3 ½ cups almond flour
2 tablespoons culinary-grade lavender
2 tablespoons lemon zest
2 tablespoons fresh lemon juice
½ teaspoon pure vanilla extract (optional)
2 tablespoons coconut oil, melted
2 tablespoons pure maple syrup

Mix together the almond flour, lavender, lemon zest and juice, vanilla, coconut oil, and maple syrup in a large bowl to create the cookie dough.

Place the entire mixture between two pieces of parchment paper and roll out the dough into ¼- to ½-inch-thick circles. Remove the top sheet of parchment and use a cookie cutter to form your cookies. Reroll the dough scraps to cut out more cookies. Place the cookies on a large plate and chill in the refrigerator to set.

✦ ✦ ✦ ✦

BEAUTY FOOD SPOTLIGHT

Lavender has long been used to treat various skin conditions, such as acne and psoriasis. The polyphenols in this soothing herb can also help reduce the bad bacteria in your gut, keeping your stomach slim and trim.

✦ ✦ ✦ ✦

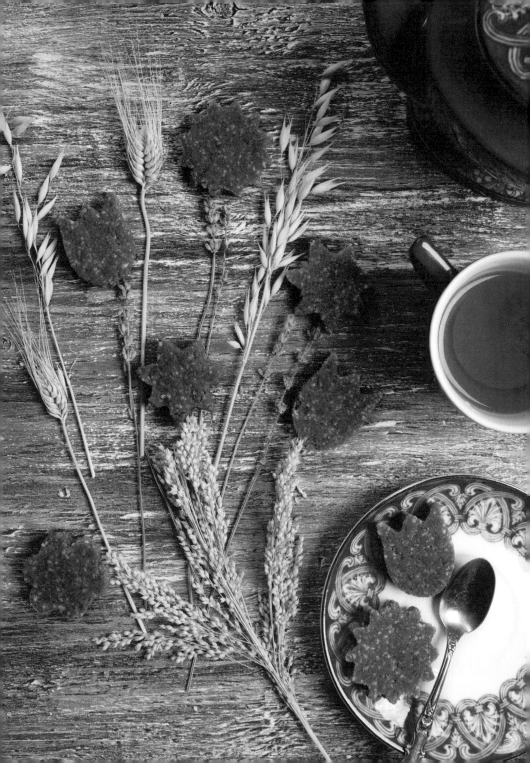

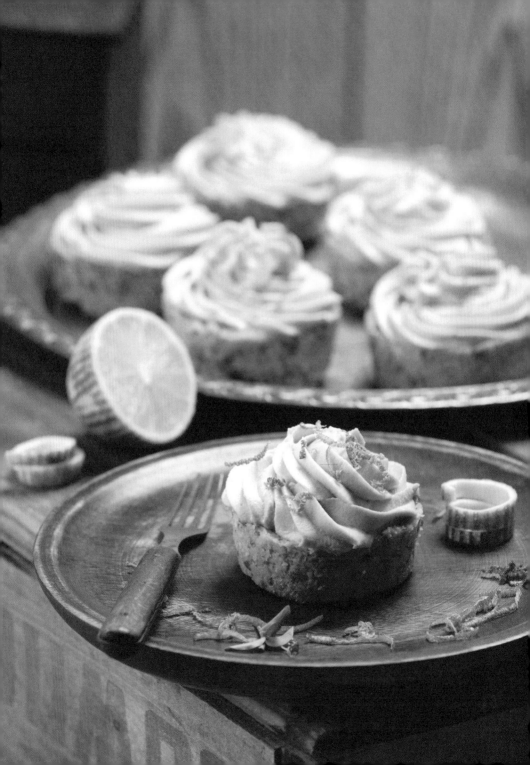

RAW MATCHA KEY LIME CUPCAKES

With a smooth, dense, and creamy texture and bright citrus notes, these deliciously sweet and zesty rounds of bliss are the utter definition of skin food. Loaded with healthy fats from the avocado, nuts, and coconut, and the added antioxidants from the matcha tea, these will keep your sweet tooth satisfied and your skin glowing.

MAKES 12 CUPCAKES

Coconut macadamia crust
2 cups raw macadamia nuts
1 cup unsweetened dried shredded coconut
1 tablespoon lime zest
2 tablespoons fresh lime juice
2 teaspoons pure vanilla extract
¼ cup pure maple syrup
1 teaspoon sea salt

Key lime filling
1½ cups raw cashews, soaked in water for 2 hours, then drained
1 avocado, halved and pitted
⅔ cups Key lime or regular lime juice
2 tablespoons pure maple syrup
1 tablespoon matcha powder (optional)
2 tablespoons lime zest, for garnish

(continued)

To make the crust:

Place all the crust ingredients in a food processor and pulse until well combined. The mixture should appear crumbly but stick together easily when pressed.

Line a twelve-well muffin pan with paper liners. Place 2 tablespoons of the dough inside each cup and flatten it against the bottom of the cup to form a crust. Repeat with the remaining mixture. Place the tray in the freezer to set and chill.

To make the Key lime filling:

Place all the filling ingredients in a food processor and process into a smooth, creamy mixture. Remove the muffin pan from the freezer and transfer the cupcake crusts to a large plate. Scoop the filling onto each cup. Garnish with lime zest. Chill before serving.

✦ ✦ ✦ ✦

BEAUTY FOOD SPOTLIGHT

Matcha contains various antioxidants and polyphenols that,
together, help boost the immune system and protect against antigens.
Chlorophyll-rich matcha is also an excellent detoxifier that cleanses the
blood, maintaining its alkalinity and flushes toxins out of the body.

✦ ✦ ✦ ✦

GOLDEN MILK ICE-CREAM BROWNIE SANDWICHES

Tucked between two chunks of these oh-so-chocolaty, nutty, chewy brownies is creamy, coconut milk-based ice cream, inspired from the sweet and spicy drink affectionately known as Golden Milk. Ground turmeric, cinnamon, black pepper, ginger, and cardamom bring plenty of rich, warm flavor to this delicious frozen treat.

SERVES 8

ICE CREAM
2 cups canned coconut milk
4 (quarter-size) slices fresh ginger
½ cup pure maple syrup
2 teaspoons ground turmeric
1 teaspoon ground cinnamon
½ teaspoon freshly ground black pepper
1 teaspoon ground cardamom
Sea salt
1 teaspoon pure vanilla extract
4 bananas, frozen

RAW BROWNIES
1½ cups walnuts
Sea salt
8 Medjool dates, pitted
⅓ cup raw cacao powder
1 teaspoon pure vanilla extract
2 teaspoons water

(continued)

To make the ice cream:

Place the coconut milk, ginger, maple syrup, turmeric, cinnamon, pepper, cardamom, and salt to taste in a large saucepan and heat over medium heat.

Bring to a simmer, whisking to combine. Remove from the heat and add the vanilla. Whisk once more.

Taste and adjust the flavor as needed, adding more turmeric for intense turmeric flavor, cinnamon for warmth, maple syrup for sweetness, or salt to balance the flavors.

Transfer the mixture to a bowl and let cool to room temperature.

Strain the mixture, transfer to a blender, add the bananas, and blend.

Transfer the mixture to a large, freezer-safe container and freeze for 2 hours. Remove from the freezer and process in the blender once more.

Cover securely and freeze overnight, until firm.

To make the brownies:

Chop ¼ cup of the walnuts and set aside. Place the remaining walnuts and salt to taste in a food processor or blender and process until finely ground. Add the dates and process until the mixture sticks together. Add the cacao powder, vanilla, and water and process to distribute. Transfer the mixture to a glass container and pack it in evenly. Spread the reserved walnuts evenly on top. Place in the refrigerator to cool. Cut into squares before serving.

To assemble the ice-cream sandwiches, cut a brownie in two horizontally and scoop ice cream between the two halves. Serve immediately.

✦   ✦   ✦   ✦

KITCHEN NOTE

Take care not to overprocess the frozen bananas, as they will melt and ruin the ice-cream effect.

✦   ✦   ✦   ✦

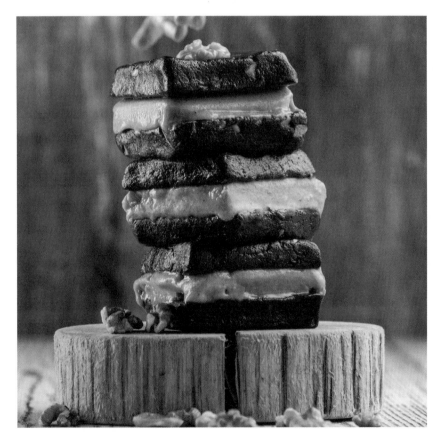

++++

BEAUTY FOOD SPOTLIGHT

Golden Milk is a truly synergistic healing blend. The turmeric and curcumin, its most documented bioactive ingredient, include powerful antioxidant, anti-inflammatory, and healing properties.
Black pepper, whose sharp taste comes from the alkaloid piperine, enhances the anti-inflammatory effects of turmeric. And since turmeric is also fat soluble, the coconut milk maximizes absorption of its healing properties.

++++

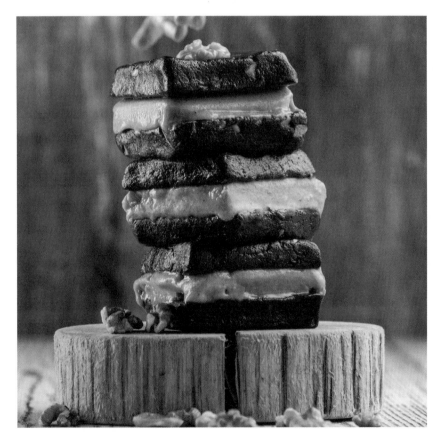

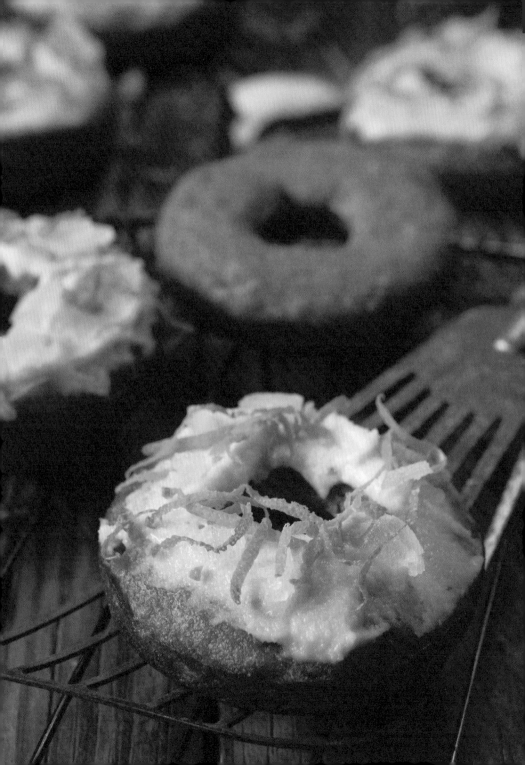

CARROT CAKE DONUTS WITH CITRUS CREAM CHEESE FROSTING

Donuts and carrot cake in one delicious, nutritious bite? Check! These sweet baked cake donuts are infused with all the moist deliciousness of carrot cake and topped with the absolutely essential citrus cream cheese frosting.

MAKES 6

DONUTS

⅓ cup coconut oil, melted and cooled, plus more for pan

¾ cup shredded carrot

2 tablespoons pure maple syrup

1 teaspoon pure vanilla extract

⅓ cup almond butter

6 tablespoons filtered water

2 tablespoons flaxseed meal

1¼ cups almond flour

1 teaspoon baking powder

½ cup walnuts (optional)

½ cup unsweetened shredded coconut (optional)

(continued)

½ cup raw cashews, soaked in water for 2 hours, then drained
Zest of 1 orange
3 tablespoons fresh orange juice
1 tablespoon pure maple syrup
1 teaspoon grated fresh ginger

To make the donuts:

Preheat the oven to 350°F. Grease a donut pan well with coconut oil.

Whisk together the ¼ cup of coconut oil, carrot, maple syrup, vanilla, and almond butter in a large bowl until well combined. Add the water, flaxseed meal, almond flour, and baking powder and mix well.

Fold in the walnuts and coconut, if using. Pour the mixture into the prepared pan and bake for 12 minutes, or until a toothpick inserted into a donut ring comes out clean.

Remove from the oven and let cool before removing from the donut pan.

To make the frosting:

Place the cashews in a blender or food processor and process. Add the rest of the frosting ingredients, reserving half of the orange zest, and blend until smooth and creamy. Transfer to a bowl and refrigerate for 10 minutes.

Using a spoon, gently spread the glaze on top of the donuts. Top with the reserved orange zest. Store the leftover frosting and donuts in separate glass containers in the refrigerator for up to 1 week. The frosting will spoil faster if on donuts, so either keep separately until ready to enjoy or enjoy within 3 days.

+ + + +

BEAUTY FOOD SPOTLIGHT

Most of the benefits of carrots can be attributed to their beta-carotene fiber and vitamin A content, keeping your eyes beautiful by promoting regenerating collagen, aiding cell division, and the slowing of eyesight deterioration.

+ + + +

MILLE CREPE CAKE WITH SALTED CRÈME CARAMEL

Something magical happens when you layer crepes into a cake. Dense, creamy, moist, and flavorful, this completely grain-free version balances your hormones and blood sugar for a flawless complexion.

SERVES 8 TO 12

Crepes
2 cup chickpea flour
3 cups almond milk
½ cup coconut oil, plus more for pan
6 tablespoons pure maple syrup
2 teaspoons pure vanilla extract
2 teaspoons ground cinnamon
1 teaspoon sea salt

Salted crème caramel
½ cup pure maple syrup
½ cup almond butter
¼ cup coconut oil
2 teaspoons pure vanilla extract
2 teaspoons orange zest
½ teaspoon sea salt

To make the crepes:
Combine the almond milk, coconut oil, maple syrup, vanilla, cinnamon, and sea salt in a large bowl. Whisk in the flour until well combined.

(continued)

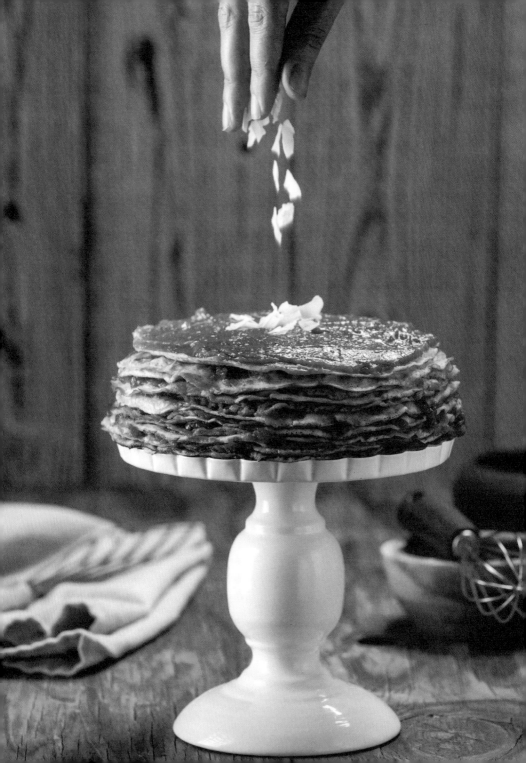

Heat a lightly greased a skillet or griddle over medium-low heat. Pour ¼ cup of the batter into the skillet and immediately rotate the pan until the batter evenly coats the bottom in a thin layer. Cook until the top of the crepe is no longer wet and the bottom has turned light brown. Run a spatula around the edge of the skillet to loosen; flip the crepe and cook until the other side has turned light brown. Repeat with the remaining batter.

To make the crème caramel:
Whisk together all the crème caramel ingredients in a small saucepan over medium-low heat until smooth, about 3 minutes. Remove from the heat and let cool slightly.

To assemble, lay a crepe on a serving plate. Using a spatula, cover with a layer of caramel sauce. Cover with a second crepe and repeat to make a stack of twenty, reserving the best-looking crepe to be placed on top. Cover with plastic wrap and chill for at least 2 hours.

Serve with an extra drizzle of crème caramel sauce.

✦ ✦ ✦ ✦

KITCHEN NOTE

For best texture and flavor, let the crepe batter sit for 15 minutes. This resting step allows the batter to relax and ensures a thin and uniform crepe that is delicate instead of chewy.

✦ ✦ ✦ ✦

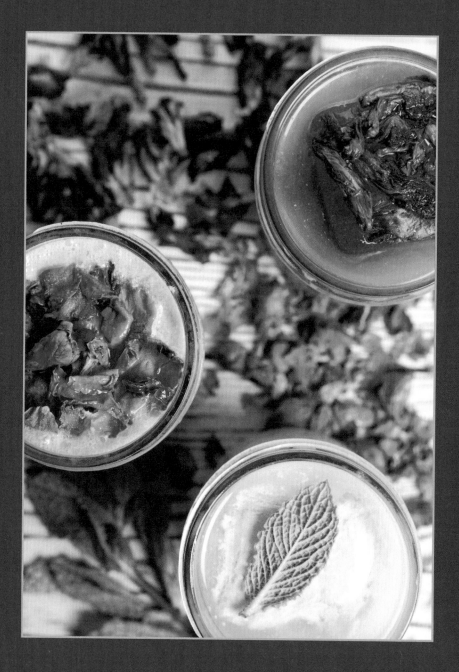

SIPPING PRETTY

Beauty Elixirs, Restorative Tonics, and Healing Lattes

Healing tonics and elixirs are an easy way to incorporate beneficial spices, roots, herbs, and botanicals into your daily ritual. From gut-healing probiotic waters to heart-opening rose lattes, the following metabolism-boosting, hormone-balancing drinks will satisfy your every mood and need.

Jeweled Rose Latte

Blue Serenity Latte

Jade Lotus Latte

Probiotic Coconut Water

Kombucha

Pomegranate Switchel

Elderberry Cordial

Marigold and Apricot Elixir

Honeysuckle Bitters

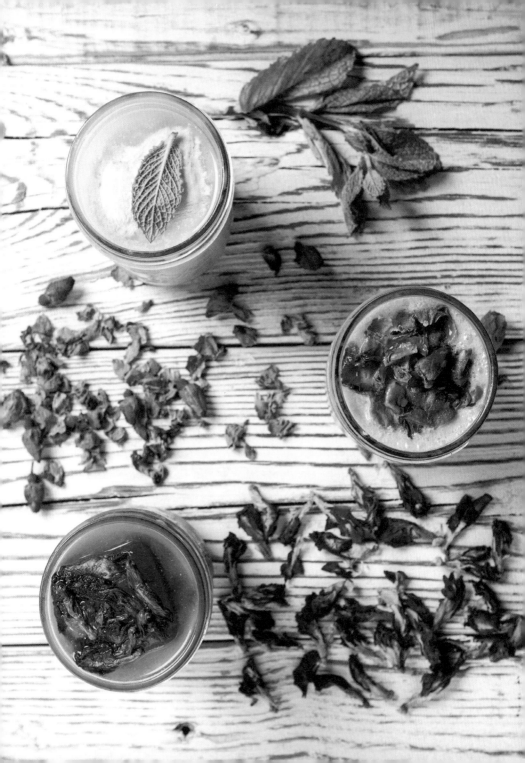

JEWELED ROSE LATTE

To be sipped and savored, this beauty elixir infuses superfood nutrients, minerals, proteins, and healthful fats into your daily ritual.

ROSE AND MAQUI BERRY SYRUP

MAKES 1 CUP

¼ cup culinary-grade dried rose petals
2 tablespoons maqui powder
1 cup filtered water
1 teaspoon rose water
1 cup pure maple syrup

PER LATTE

MAKES 1 SERVING

1 cup pistachio milk
2 tablespoons rose and maqui berry syrup
1 teaspoon maca powder (optional)

To make the rose and maqui berry syrup:
Combine all the ingredients for the syrup in a small saucepan over medium-high heat. Simmer, stirring frequently, until the maple syrup and powder have fully dissolved. Remove from the heat and let steep for 15 minutes. Pour through a fine-mesh strainer, pressing the dried flowers to get out all the liquid. Transfer to a clean jar, cover, and keep refrigerated for up to 2 weeks.

(continued)

To make the latte:

Mix all the latte ingredients in a high-speed blender for 1 to 2 minutes, until well blended. Serve warm and frothy.

✦ ✦ ✦ ✦

BEAUTY FOOD SPOTLIGHT

With an abundance of B vitamins and vitamins A, C, and E, rose water can lighten dark spots, tighten pores, and keep skin well hydrated and healthy looking.

✦ ✦ ✦ ✦

BLUE SERENITY LATTE

LAVENDER AND BUTTERFLY PEA SYRUP

MAKES 1 CUP

¼ cup dried culinary-grade pea flowers
¼ cup culinary-grade lavender buds
1 cup filtered water
1 cup pure maple syrup

PER LATTE

MAKES 1 SERVING

1 cup macadamia milk
2 tablespoons lavender and butterfly pea syrup
1 teaspoon kava (optional)

To make the lavender and butterfly pea syrup:
Combine all the syrup ingredients in a small saucepan over medium-high heat. Simmer, stirring frequently, until the maple syrup has fully dissolved. Remove from the heat and let steep for 15 minutes. Pour through a fine-mesh strainer, pressing the dried flowers to get out all the liquid. Transfer to a clean jar, cover, and keep refrigerated for up to 2 weeks.

(continued)

To make the latte:

Mix all the latte ingredients in a high-speed blender for 1 to 2 minutes, until well blended. Serve warm and frothy.

❖ ❖ ❖ ❖

BEAUTY FOOD SPOTLIGHT

Kava, a.k.a. kava-kava, is a root found on South Pacific islands. Islanders have used kava as medicine and in ceremonies for centuries. Kava has a calming effect that may relieve anxiety and sleeplessness. Sipping a kava drink is an excellent way to preserve and maintain collagen levels that keep skin tight and your complexion bright. Traditionally prepared as a tea, kava root is easy to use as a powder or tincture. Use in creamy, high-fat-content drinks to mask its strong, chalky, bitter taste.

❖ ❖ ❖ ❖

JADE LOTUS LATTE

VANILLA JASMINE SYRUP

MAKES 1 CUP

2 vanilla beans
¼ cup culinary-grade dried jasmine buds
1 cup filtered water
1 cup pure maple syrup

PER LATTE

MAKES 1 SERVING

1 cup cashew milk
2 tablespoons vanilla jasmine syrup
1 teaspoon matcha

To make the vanilla jasmine syrup:
Slit each vanilla bean gently down the middle and scrape out the black seeds. Place the seeds and pod in a small saucepan over medium-high heat along with the remaining syrup ingredients. Simmer, stirring frequently, until the maple syrup has fully dissolved. Remove from the heat and let steep for 15 minutes. Pour through a fine-mesh strainer, pressing the dried flowers to get out all the liquid. Transfer to a clean jar, cover, and keep refrigerated for up to 2 weeks.

(continued)

To make the latte:

Mix all the latte ingredients in a high-speed blender for 1 to 2 minutes, until well blended. Serve warm and frothy.

✦ ✦ ✦ ✦

BEAUTY FOOD SPOTLIGHT

Beyond its intoxicating aroma and its soothing, relaxing effect, jasmine's high levels of catechins can accelerate the metabolism and trigger the body to burn more calories.

✦ ✦ ✦ ✦

PROBIOTIC COCONUT WATER

One of the main functions of healthful bacteria is to stimulate immune response. Surprisingly, 80 percent of our immune system is located in our digestive tract. By eating and drinking probiotic-rich foods and maintaining good intestinal flora, we can naturally boost our immunity and overall beauty.

A rich probiotic drink loaded with vitamins, minerals, and electrolytes, probiotic coconut water destroys pathogenic yeasts in the body and clears dull skin.

MAKES 2 CUPS

2 cups raw coconut water
1 teaspoon probiotics

Pour the coconut water into a glass container and mix in the probiotics. Cover the jar with cheesecloth. Keep in a warm place in your kitchen for 24 to 48 hours.

Store in an airtight container in the refrigerator for up to 3 days.

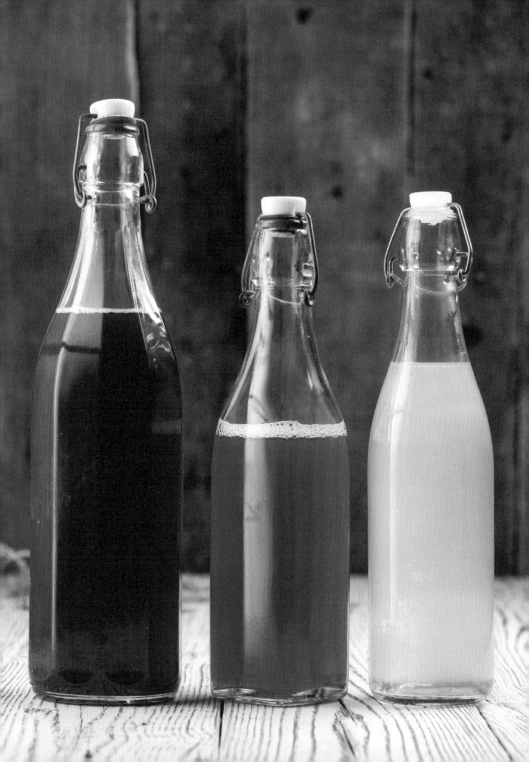

KOMBUCHA

A naturally carbonated, fermented tea drink packed with enzymes, probiotics, and beneficial acids, kombucha detoxifies, hydrates, and improves skin elasticity. Make it at home for less than half the price of store-bought. This recipe is for 1 gallon. Scale up or down to make as much as you need.

MAKES 1 GALLON

1 gallon water
8 green or black tea bags
1 cup coconut sugar
1 scoby (kombucha starter)

Bring ½ gallon of the water to a boil in a large pot. Add the tea bags and allow to steep for 20 minutes. Remove the tea bags. Add the sugar and stir well. Allow the tea to come to room temperature and pour into a clean 1-gallon glass jar. Add the remaining ½ gallon of water to the jar and place the scoby in the jar. Cover with cheesecloth and secure with a rubber band. Allow the kombucha to ferment in a dark place for 1 to 2 weeks.

✦ ✦ ✦ ✦

KITCHEN NOTE

*Made by crystallizing sap from the coconut palm tree, coconut sugar
is rich in minerals. The mineral content may require a shorter
brewing cycle. Taste frequently to find the right brewing cycle length
for your taste preferences.*

✦ ✦ ✦ ✦

POMEGRANATE SWITCHEL

A switchel is a combination of molasses, vinegar, and ginger. Together, these sweet, tangy, and spicy ingredients provide valuable minerals and electrolytes that work to improve your digestion, reduce bloating, and clear up your skin.

Pomegranate molasses
MAKES 2 CUPS

2 cups pomegranate juice
1 tablespoon fresh lemon juice
½ cup pure maple syrup

Per switchel
MAKES 1 CUP

2 tablespoons pomegranate molasses
1 tablespoon raw apple cider vinegar
1 teaspoon grated fresh ginger
1 cup water

To make the pomegranate molasses:
Combine the pomegranate juice, lemon juice, and maple syrup in a saucepan over medium-low heat. Simmer, stirring frequently, for 30 minutes. Remove from the heat and let cool. The molasses will continue to thicken as it cools. Store in the refrigerator for up to 1 month.

To make the switchel:
Combine all the switchel ingredients, except the water, in a glass jar and stir until the molasses has dissolved. Add the water and stir to combine.

Cover and refrigerate overnight. Infuse longer for a stronger ginger flavor. Strain and discard the solids.

ELDERBERRY CORDIAL

Elderberries, of the genus *Sambucus*, have long been used in medicinal tonics and cordials. The bioflavonoids in elderberries, combined with their vitamin A content, help prevent skin from premature aging and generally improve the glow and tone of your skin.

MAKES 3 CUPS

1¼ cups dried elderberries
2 tablespoons dried orange peel
Approximately 3 cups brandy
Pure maple syrup

Combine the elderberries and orange peel in a quart-size glass jar. Add brandy to fill the jar, plus maple syrup to taste, and seal. Set aside in a cool, dark place for 3 to 4 weeks.

Strain through cheesecloth over a large bowl. Bottle and store in a cool, dry place for up to 1 year.

✦　✦　✦　✦

KITCHEN NOTE

Infusions involve steeping herbs, roots, flowers, spices, or fruits in alcohol to preserve and extract their powerful herbal properties. Elixirs, liqueurs, and cordials are sweet; bitters, made from bitter herbs, are well, bitter. Here are a few recipes to get you started.

✦　✦　✦　✦

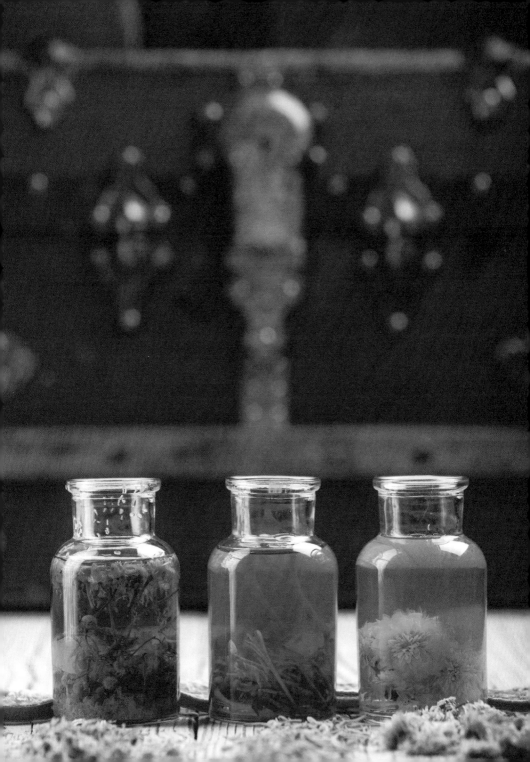

MARIGOLD AND APRICOT ELIXIR

Marigold, also known as calendula, has been used medicinally for centuries. With its high content of flavonoids, calendula has regenerative properties that can help hair grow faster and stronger.

MAKES 3 CUPS

1 cup diced dried apricots
½ cup culinary-grade dried marigolds
1 cup coconut sugar
1 medium orange, seeded and diced
3 cups vodka

Place all the ingredients into a quart-size jar. Seal and shake twice a day for 1 week. Strain the mixture through cheesecloth. Bottle and store in a cool, dry place for up to 1 year.

HONEYSUCKLE BITTERS

Sweet, grassy honeysuckle gives these digestive bitters a decisively herbaceous flavor profile. Bitters taken fifteen minutes before mealtime stimulate digestion and keep you bloat free. Try these in your next gin cocktail, spa water, or jam for a truly sublime flavor experience.

MAKES 3 CUPS

¼ cup culinary-grade dried honeysuckle flowers
1 tablespoon raw artichoke leaves
1 tablespoon cardamom seeds, cracked
2 medium oranges, seeded and diced
3 cups vodka

Place all the ingredients into a quart-size jar. Seal and shake twice a day for 1 week. Strain the mixture through cheesecloth. Bottle and store in a cool, dry place for up to 1 year.

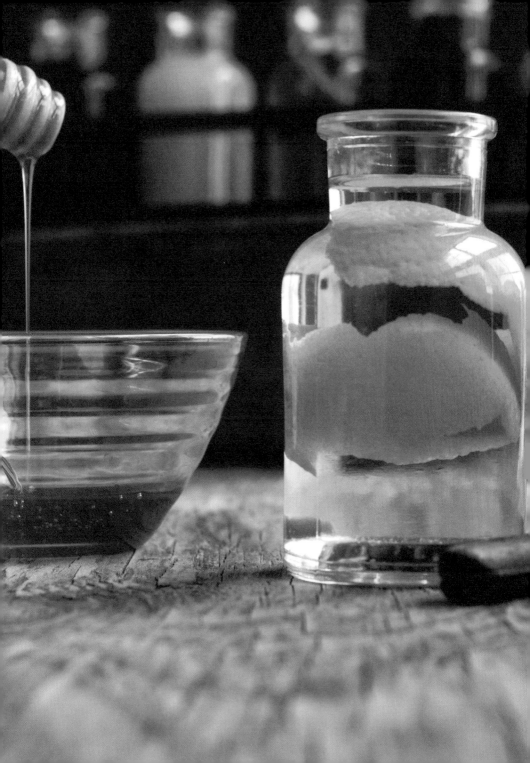

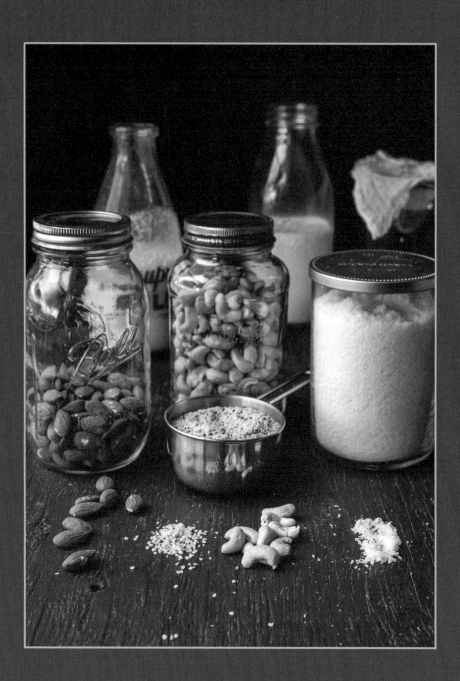

HOMEMADE PROVISIONS

Pickles, Preserves, Tasty Condiments, and Dairy-Free Substitutes

A tasty marinara sauce can elevate your humble plate of pasta just like a hot sauce can make or break your bowl of chili. Condiments and pantry staples bring zest to your dishes and are as easy as whipping up a few ingredients in your blender. The following recipes are for those can't-live-without condiments, pickles, and preserves minus the extra ingredients that wreck havoc on our skin and bellies.

Plus, all the creamy dairy-free staples that will keep your tummy happy and bloat free.

Nut and Seed Milks

Basic Vegan Cheeses

Yogurts and Spreads

Condiments and Seasonings

Pickles and Ferments

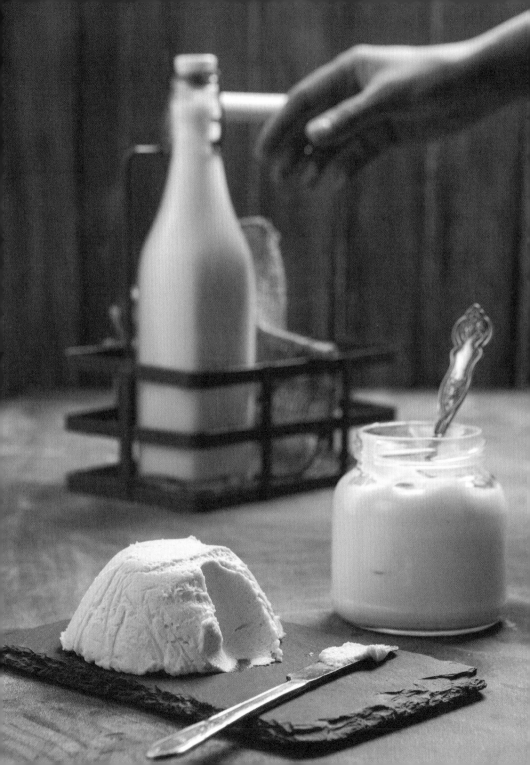

NUT AND SEED MILKS

Nut and seed milks are easy to make at home, and best of all, you'll avoid the sweeteners, thickeners, emulsifiers, stabilizers, and preservatives added to commercial versions. Simply blended with water, many types of nuts and seeds transform into a deliciously creamy milk alternative.

NUT OR SEED MILK MASTER RECIPE

This basic recipe works with most nuts or seeds. Store for up to three to five days in the refrigerator. If the milk separates, shake or blend again before using.

Soak the nuts or seeds following the appropriate soaking times in the table. Besides yielding a creamier milk, soaking releases enzyme inhibitors that make it easier to digest. Strain the soaked nuts or seeds and rinse well.

Nut/Seed	Quantity	Water (filtered/purified)	Soaking Time
Almonds	1 cup	3 cups	8 hours
Brazil nuts	1 cup	3 cups	6 hours
Cashews	1 cup	3 cups	6 hours
Macadamias	1 cup	3 cups	6 hours
Hazelnuts	1 cup	2 cups	8–10 hours
Flaxseeds	¼ cup	3 cups	1 hour
Sunflower seeds	1 cup	3 cups	8 hours
Hemp seeds	½ cup	4 cups	No soaking necessary

Place the nuts or the seeds in a blender, add the measured water (see chart), and process until smooth. Use a fine-mesh strainer, cheesecloth, or nut milk bag to strain out any particles.

VARIATIONS: For creams, reduce the water by half; for skim milks, add more water.

Tasty Tweaks: Customize the flavor of nut and seed milks with these tasty add-ins:

Vanilla Milk: Add 1 tablespoon of pure vanilla extract and blend with one or two pitted dates or your preferred natural sweetener.

Chocolate Milk: Add 1 tablespoon of raw cacao powder and sweeten with organic agave or pure maple syrup. Use hazelnuts for an extra special Nutella-like milk!

Strawberry Rose Milk: Blend in 1 cup of fresh or frozen strawberries and add 2 teaspoons of pure rose water.

Carrot Cake Milk: Blend in 2 chopped medium carrots, 1 teaspoon of pure vanilla extract, 1½ teaspoons of ground cinnamon, and ¼ teaspoon of ground cardamom. Sweeten to taste with maple syrup.

Chai Milk: Add ½ teaspoon of ground cardamom, ¼ teaspoon of ground cinnamon, two peppercorns, and three thin slivers of fresh ginger. Sweeten with dates or maple syrup to taste.

Matcha Milk: Add 1½ teaspoons of matcha green tea powder and sweeten to taste with maple syrup.

✦　✦　✦　✦

KITCHEN NOTE

If you don't want the hassle of straining out nut pulp, you'll love working with cashews. Just soak, drain, rinse, and blend with water for an ever-so-creamy milk with no pulp left behind.

✦　✦　✦　✦

COCONUT MILK

Making your own coconut milk is a pure delight. If you have access to young coconuts, I encourage you to try your hand at this lovely milk alternative. Nothing like the overly processed and sweetened coconut beverages, home-made coconut milk is very low in calories and has tremendous health benefits.

MAKES 2 TO 3 CUPS OF COCONUT MILK

1 to 2 young Thai coconuts

Remove all the meat and water from the coconut shells. Rinse the coconut meat and place the meat and water in a blender. Blend until smooth. Strain the mixture to remove any small shell particles.

✦ ✦ ✦ ✦

KITCHEN NOTE

Hate to throw away the blended pulp used for milk? Add it to smoothies to boost protein and fiber or turn into a meal or flour, for use in cookies, crusts, and crackers.

✦ ✦ ✦ ✦

How to Make a Nut Flour

Store-bought coconut and almond flours can be quite pricey. Making your own from the strained solids of your nut milks, however, is quite simple. Pour the strained-out solids onto a parchment-lined baking sheet and bake in a 250°F oven for 2 to 3 hours. Transfer to a blender and process into a flour. The flour will keep refrigerated for up to 5 days.

Quick Milk

In a hurry or not in the mood to make a traditional nut milk?
This quick version is all you need:

3¾ cups filtered water
1 cup almond meal or flour
2 to 3 Medjool dates, pitted
½ teaspoon pure vanilla extract
¼ teaspoon sea salt

Place all the ingredients in a blender and blend until smooth.
Use as a substitute for regular nut milk in recipes or enjoy as is.
Store in an airtight glass container in the refrigerator for
up to 3 to 4 days.

BASIC VEGAN CHEESES

CHEESE SPREAD

This simple spread is remarkably quick and easy to make and is perfect to have on hand as a basic creamy cheese spread.

MAKES ABOUT 1 CUP

1 cup raw cashews, soaked in water for 2 hours, then drained
2 tablespoons fresh lemon juice
2 to 3 tablespoons water
2 tablespoons nutritional yeast
½ teaspoon sea salt

Place the cashews in a blender along with the water, lemon juice, nutritional yeast, and salt and blend until smooth. Transfer the cheese to a bowl and allow to set and chill in the refrigerator for at least 1 hour.

Will keep in a covered container in the refrigerator for up to 1 week.

For many more dairy-free cheese options, both hard and soft, and meltable, spreadable, and sliceable, please check out my book *Vegan Cheese: Simple, Delicious, Plant-Based Recipes*.

NUT OR SEED PARMESAN

Here's your almost instant dairy-free solution to the cheesy sprinkle.

MAKES I CUP

1 cup raw seeds or nuts
½ cup nutritional yeast
Sea salt and freshly ground black pepper

Place all the ingredients, including salt and pepper to taste, in a food processor or a coffee or nut grinder and pulse until the texture resembles that of finely grated Parmesan.

Transfer to an airtight glass jar. Store in the refrigerator for up to 1 month.

Interested in more sophisticated vegan cheese recipes?
Check out my book
Vegan Cheese: Simple, Delicious, Plant-Based Recipes.

YOGURTS AND SPREADS

These probiotic-rich, creamy yogurt recipes are simple to master. Try them both to find your favorite.

CASHEW YOGURT

MAKES 2 CUPS

2 cups cashews, soaked in water for 8 hours or overnight,
then rinsed and drained
1 teaspoon probiotic powder
Filtered water
1 tablespoon raw apple cider vinegar
Sea salt

Place the cashews and probiotic in a high-speed blender and blend to a smooth consistency, adding filtered water, 1 tablespoon at a time, as needed. Transfer the mixture to a glass container and cover with cheesecloth. Keep in a warm place in your kitchen for 12 hours.

Transfer the yogurt to a blender, add the vinegar and salt, and blend. Pour the yogurt back into a glass container, cover with cheesecloth, and chill in the refrigerator for another 12 hours.

Store in an airtight container in the refrigerator for up to 5 days.

You may need to experiment with the length of time of the yogurt cultures and with the amount of probiotic you use. Everyone has different taste preferences and experimenting will allow you to customize your yogurt to your taste.

COCONUT YOGURT

2 cups coconut meat
1 cup coconut water
2 tablespoons fresh lemon juice
½ teaspoon sea salt
1 teaspoon probiotic powder

Combine the coconut meat, coconut water, lemon juice, salt, and probiotics in a blender and blend until smooth. Transfer the mixture to a glass jar and cover the jar with cheesecloth.

Keep in a warm place in your kitchen for 12 hours. After 8 hours, the yogurt should thicken and taste slightly tart. If you prefer a tarter taste, leave the yogurt for another 4 hours. Store in an airtight container in the refrigerator for up to 5 days.

SOUR CREAM

You can feel good about this dairy-free, protein- and mineral-rich cashew–based spin on sour cream.

MAKES 1½ CUPS

1 cup raw cashews, soaked in water for 8 hours, then drained
½ to ¾ cup filtered water
2 tablespoons fresh lemon juice
1 tablespoon raw apple cider vinegar
Sea salt

Place all the ingredients, including salt to taste, in a blender and blend until smooth. Transfer to an airtight glass jar. Store in the refrigerator for up to 4 days.

SWEET CREAM

A sweet nondairy cream to adorn your favorite desserts and chia puddings.

MAKES 1½ CUPS

1 cup raw cashews, soaked in water for 2 hours, then drained
½ cup filtered water
2 Medjool dates, pitted
Pinch of salt

Place all the ingredients in a blender and blend until smooth. Transfer to an airtight glass jar. Store in the refrigerator for up to 4 days.

GARLIC AND DILL BUTTERY SPREAD

This creamy spread is reminiscent of the herbed garlic butter served at the finest restaurants, but is the all-natural, plant-based version.

MAKES 2 CUPS

2 cups raw cashews, soaked in water for 2 hours, then drained
1 cup coconut oil, melted
2 tablespoons minced fresh dill
1 teaspoon garlic powder
Sea salt and freshly ground black pepper

Place all the ingredients in a food processor or blender and process until smooth. Transfer to an airtight glass jar. Store in the refrigerator for up to 1 week.

CONDIMENTS AND SEASONINGS

AVO MAYO

This deliciously, creamy, plant-based, cholesterol-free version of traditional mayonnaise is packed with protein, beautifying fats, and minerals.

MAKES 2 CUPS

1 cup cashew nuts, soaked in water for 2 hours, then drained
1 avocado, peeled and pitted
¼ cup fresh lemon juice
½ cup olive oil
½ cup filtered water
1 teaspoon nutritional yeast
1 teaspoon dry mustard
2 teaspoons sea salt

Place all the ingredients in a blender and blend until smooth. Transfer to an airtight glass jar. Store in the refrigerator for up to 1 week.

BBQ SAUCE

There's nothing quite like a sweet and tangy BBQ sauce. Unless it's this homemade antioxidant-rich and flavorful version.

MAKES 3½ CUPS

2 cups filtered water
2 cups sun-dried tomatoes, soaked in water for 1 hour
2 tablespoons raw apple cider vinegar
2 tablespoons chipotle peppers in adobo sauce, seeded
1 cup olive oil
2 tablespoons tamari (or coconut aminos, for a soy-free option)
2 tablespoons pure maple syrup
2 tablespoons blackstrap molasses
1 teaspoon onion powder
1 teaspoon garlic powder
½ teaspoon ground allspice
Sea salt and freshly ground black pepper

Place all the ingredients, including salt and pepper to taste, in a blender and blend until smooth. Transfer to an airtight glass jar. Store in the refrigerator for up to 1 week.

KETCHUP

Everybody's favorite condiment, packed with fresh, antioxidant-rich ingredients minus the artificial additives.

MAKES ABOUT 1½ CUPS

½ cup peeled and diced red onion
3 garlic cloves, peeled and crushed
2 cups roughly chopped tomato
1 tablespoon pure maple syrup
3 tablespoon raw apple cider vinegar
1 tablespoon umeboshi plum vinegar (optional)
Sea salt and freshly ground black pepper

Place the onion and garlic in a saucepan over medium heat and cook for 4 minutes, or until soft. Lower the heat to low and add the tomato. Simmer for 8 minutes, stirring frequently, or until the tomatoes begin to break down and soften. Add the remaining ingredients, except the plum vinegar, and including salt and pepper to taste, and mash the tomato, using a wooden spoon. Simmer for an additional 15 minutes.

Remove from the heat and let cool.

Transfer to a blender, add the plum vinegar if using, and blend until smooth. Taste and adjust the seasoning to your preference. Transfer to an airtight glass jar. Store in the refrigerator for up to 1 week.

HARISSA

Enjoy making this traditional North African chili sauce at home without the need for artificial preservatives.

MAKES I CUP

½ cup olive oil
2 red bell peppers, seeded and deveined
2 garlic cloves, peeled and crushed
2 tablespoons paprika
3 tablespoons fresh lemon juice
2 tablespoons pure maple syrup
1 tablespoon red pepper flakes
1 tablespoon ground cumin
1 teaspoon ground coriander
Sea salt and freshly ground black pepper

Place all the ingredients, including salt and pepper to taste, in a blender and blend until smooth. Transfer to an airtight glass jar. Store in the refrigerator for up to 2 weeks.

ZA'ATAR

A Middle Eastern spice blend comprising toasted sesame seeds, sumac, cumin, and dried herbs.

MAKES ¼ CUP

1 tablespoon sesame seeds
1 tablespoon ground sumac
1 teaspoon dried cumin
1 teaspoon dried oregano
1 teaspoon dried thyme
1 teaspoon dried mint
1 teaspoon sea salt

Combine all the ingredients in a spice grinder and grind to a coarse powder. Transfer to a sealed container.

SUPERFOOD SEASONING

This easy-to-make mixture is completely customizable and makes seasoning your meals simple and nutritious. Mix together your herbs, spices, and seeds, then generously sprinkle the goodness over your soups, snacks, salads, and entrées.

MAKES 1½ CUPS

¼ cup kelp flakes
¼ cup flaxseed meal
¼ cup nutritional yeast
¼ cup dried parsley
¼ cup dried thyme
¼ cup nettle flakes
¼ cup red pepper flakes

ADDITIONAL ADD-INS (OPTIONAL)
¼ cup dried sage
¼ cup celery seeds
¼ cup dill seeds
¼ cup hemp seeds
¼ cup sesame seeds
¼ cup sunflower seeds

Mix together all the ingredients in a medium bowl and transfer to an airtight glass jar. Store in a cool, dark spot for up to 1 month.

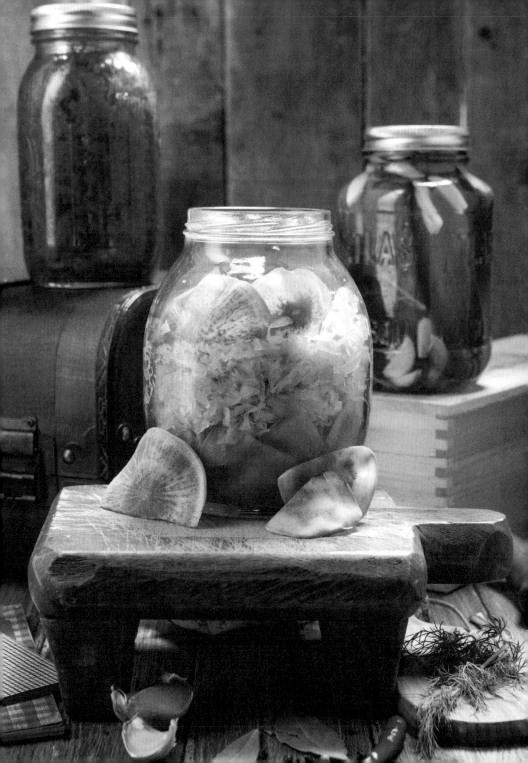

PICKLES AND FERMENTS

One of the best ways to boost the healthy bacteria in your gut is to increase your intake of fermented foods. Raw sauerkraut, kimchi, brined pickles, kombucha, and probiotic or kefir waters develop these bacteria during the fermentation process.

Try adding a serving of fermented veggies to your diet to nourish a healthy gut and to support radiant skin and fewer allergies. Here are three different recipes to experiment with.

For fermented drink recipes, please see pages 183–186.

PURPLE KIMCHI

MAKES 1 QUART

1 red cabbage, shredded
1 tablespoon kosher salt
1 tablespoon minced garlic
2 teaspoons red pepper flakes
1 tablespoon minced fresh ginger
Filtered water
1 cup shredded daikon
1 cup shredded carrot
¼ cup finely slivered scallion

Place the shredded red cabbage and salt in a large bowl. Using your hands, massage the salt into the cabbage for 5 to 10 minutes, until it starts to soften and release juices.

In a separate small bowl, combine the garlic, ginger, red pepper flakes, and 3 tablespoons of filtered water and mix to form a smooth paste.

(continued)

Add the daikon, carrots, scallion, and kimchi paste to the shredded cabbage. Using your hands, gently massage the paste into the vegetables until they are thoroughly coated.

Transfer the seasoned vegetables, including any liquid, to a quart-size jar, pressing down on the mixture until the brine rises to cover the vegetables. Leave at least 1 inch of headspace before sealing the jar. Let the jar stand at room temperature for 4 to 5 days.

Check the kimchi once a day, pressing down on the vegetables with a wooden spoon to help release the gases produced during fermentation. Refrigerate after 4 to 5 days.

SPICY CULTURED APPLE SLAW

MAKES 1 QUART

1 medium green cabbage, shredded

1 tablespoon sea salt

Filtered water

2 green apples, cored and shredded

4 jalapeño peppers, seeded

Juice of 2 limes

2 garlic cloves

2 teaspoons juniper berries

2 watermelon radishes or radishes of your choice, sliced thinly

Place the cabbage and salt in a large bowl. Using your hands, massage the salt into the cabbage for 5 to 10 minutes, until it starts to soften and release juices.

Add the apples, jalapeños, lime juice, garlic, and juniper berries to the shredded cabbage. Using your hands, gently massage the fruit and vegetables.

Line the bottom of a quart-size jar with radish slices and transfer the seasoned vegetables—including any liquid to the jar—pressing down on it until the brine rises to cover the vegetables. Place the remaining radish slices at the top, leaving at least 1 inch of headspace before sealing the jar. Let the jar stand at room temperature for 4 to 5 days.

Check the slaw once a day, pressing down on the vegetables with a wooden spoon to help release the gases produced during fermentation. Refrigerate after 4 to 5 days.

GARLIC DILL PICKLES

MAKES 1 QUART

10 Persian cucumbers
1 tablespoon chopped garlic
1 red chile pepper, seeded and halved
½ cup chopped fresh dill

BRINE

2 tablespoons sea salt
4 cups water
1 tablespoon whole peppercorns
4 bay leaves
1 tablespoon raw apple cider vinegar

Place the cucumbers in a quart-size jar and add the garlic, chile pepper, and fresh dill.

To make the brine:
Combine the brine ingredients in a saucepan over medium heat and bring to a boil. Remove from the heat and let cool for 5 minutes. Pour the brine into the jar, covering the cucumber completely. Cover and let stand at room temperature in a cool, dark place for 3 days. Check on the pickles daily to make sure they stay submerged in the brine. Refrigerate after 3 days.

✦   ✦   ✦   ✦

KITCHEN NOTE

Make sure your pickles and ferments are cured in a salt brine, not vinegar like most kinds you find in the grocery aisle, to ensure that they contain good probiotic bacteria.

✦   ✦   ✦   ✦

RESOURCES AND FURTHER READING

JulesAron.com: For the most up-to-date beauty and wellness news, recipes, products, and inspiration. Visit the site to arrange a personal consultation or to find out about workshops, cooking classes, and online programs.

INGREDIENTS

Amazon: Almost any shelf-stable ingredient or kitchen tool you can't find locally

Bob's Red Mill: Dry pantry goods, including grains, flours, and lentils

Bragg: Raw apple cider vinegar, oils, dressings

Lotus Foods: Heirloom and specialty rice and whole grains

Eden Foods: Natural and organic food line specializing in seaweed products, BPA-free canned goods, and umeboshi vinegar

Frontier Natural Products Co-op: Herbs and spices

Flower Power: Herbs and roots

Nuts.com: Nuts and seeds

Siricoco.com: Fresh coconuts and coconut water

HERBS, SUPERFOODS, AND SUPPLEMENTS

Anima Mundi Herbals: herbs, elixirs, and tonics
Herb Pharm: liquid, powdered, and topical herbs
Gaia Herbs: liquid herbal extracts
Mountain Rose Herbs: herbs, spices, teas, and DIY supplies
Navitas Naturals: organic, nutrient-dense superfood powders. Quality
    source for your pomegranate, acai, matcha, and camu-camu powders
Root & Bones: quality extracts of adaptogenic herbs and medicinal
    mushrooms
Sun Potion: superfood, tonic herbs, algaes, and skin food powders

KITCHEN TOOLS

Brevilleusa.com
Chefsresource.com
OXO.com
Vitamix.com
Williams-sonoma.com

INFORMATIONAL WEBSITES

Environmental Working Group's Cosmetics Database
Institute for Integrative Nutrition
Forks over Knives
Personalized Lifestyle Medicine Institute
Healing Spirits Herb Farm and Education Center
Traditional Chinese Medicine World Foundation

FURTHER READING

Aron, Jules. *Fresh & Pure, Organically Crafted Beauty Balms & Cleansers.* New York: The Countryman Press, 2018.

_____. *Vegan Cheese: Simple, Delicious, Plant-Based Recipes.* New York: The Countryman Press, 2017.

_____. *Zen and Tonic: Savory and Fresh Cocktails for the Enlightened Drinker.* New York: The Countryman Press, 2017.

Bittman, Mark. *Food Matters: Guide to Conscious Eating with More Than 75 Recipes.* New York: Simon & Schuster, 2009.

Drayer, Lisa. *The Beauty Diet: Looking Great Has Never Been So Delicious.* New York: McGraw-Hill, 2009.

Hart, Jolene. *Eat Pretty: Nutrition for Beauty, Inside and Out.* San Francisco: Chronicle Books, 2014.

Nestle, Marion. *Food Politics: How the Food Industry Influences Nutrition and Health.* Berkeley: University of California Press, 2013.

Pitchford, Paul. *Healing with Whole Foods: Asian Traditions and Modern Nutrition.* Berkeley: North Atlantic Books, 1993.

Pollan, Michael. *In Defense of Food: An Eater's Manifesto.* New York: Penguin Books, 2009.

Nhat Hanh, Thich. *Savor: Mindful Eating, Mindful Life.* New York: HarperOne, 2011.

Welch, Claudia. *Balance Your Hormones, Balance Your Life: Achieving Optimal Health and Wellness Through Ayurveda, Chinese Medicine, and Western Science.* Cambridge, MA: Da Capo Press, 2011.

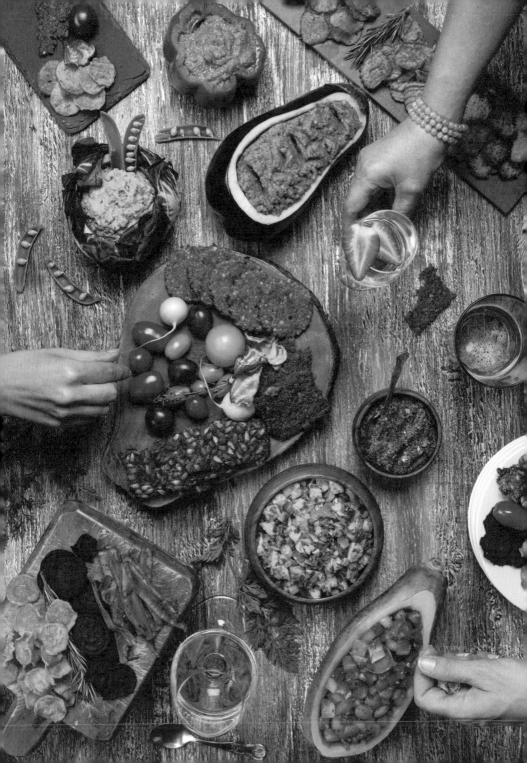

ACKNOWLEDGMENTS

The Pretty Zen collection marks my third and fourth books to date, and I am infinitely grateful for the tremendous opportunity to share these pages with so many of you beautiful souls. To the readers around the world who have been so passionately enjoying, supporting, and sharing my books, I thank you, first and foremost. May you find inspiration and guidance in these pages to fill your life with endless beauty.

It takes a group of masterful folks to produce beautiful books, and I have been lucky to have the same incredible team, give or take a few, throughout this journey.

Immeasurable gratitude:
To my literary agent, Marilyn Allen, always encouraging. Always supporting. Thank you, Marilyn, for believing in me. Your warmth and ongoing guidance mean everything to me.

To my editor extraordinaire, Ann Treistman, for your sharp and unwavering style. Thank you for your confidence in me and in my words.

To Gyorgy Papp for making my recipes come alive with your photographs. Thank you for bringing my creative vision to life.

To The Countryman Press team: Iris Bass for your thorough and capable care of my words; Aurora Bell for your unwavering grace and support; Steve Attardo, Devon Zahn, Anna Reich, and Jessica Murphy for your design and production talents; Jill Browning for your savvy marketing efforts. I am beyond grateful for all of your incredible talents. I thank you all for your time and effort.

And to my dear friends and family: Your tremendous support and amazing presence in my life is what makes this life a truly beautiful one. You are forever loved.

INDEX

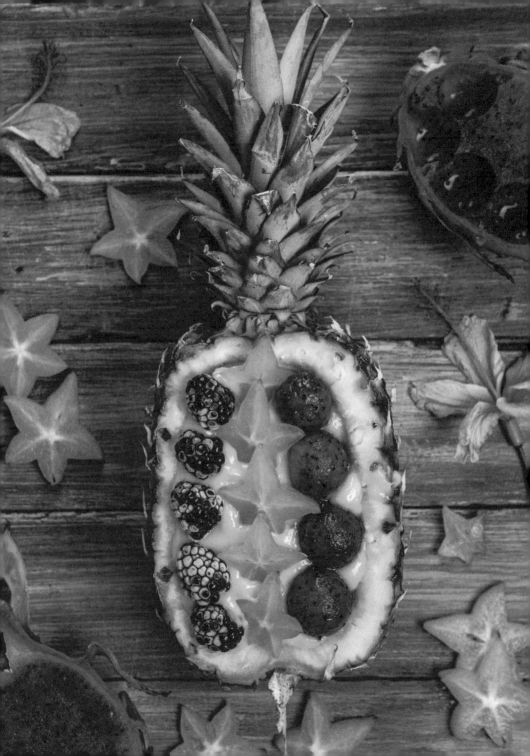

ABOUT THE AUTHOR

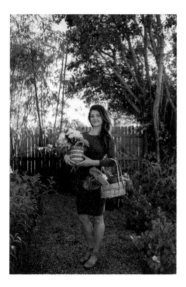

Jules Aron is a four-time best-selling author, holistic health and wellness coach, and green lifestyle expert. She is deeply passionate about a healthy, wholesome lifestyle that includes delicious, nutritious foods that fuel the body, mind, and spirit.

Jules holds a master's degree from New York University; received certification as a health and nutrition coach from the Institute of Integrative Nutrition; and is a certified yoga, qigong, and Traditional Chinese Medicine practitioner.

She is a sought-after wellness expert who has been featured in the *New York Post*, NBC News, TheTodayShow.com, *Thrive Magazine*, *Well + Good NYC*, and *Mind Body Green*. She is also a regular contributor to *Woman's World* magazine, as well as many other national media outlets.